PRAISE FOR GET TH

"*Get the Func Out* is an essential read for anyone interested in hormonal health and well-being. Dr. Kozlowski explains the functional medicine approach to hormone balance, especially its relationship to hidden environmental toxins. I can't recommend this book highly enough."

—JOEL M. EVANS, MD, *Board Certified OB/GYN, Director, The Center for Functional Medicine, Stamford, CT*

"I always focus on lowering my patient's toxic load when they present with hormonal imbalances. *Get the Func Out* does a great job at explaining the connection between toxins and your hormones and most importantly how to lower your toxic load and help rebalance your hormones."

—ELIZABETH BOHAM, MD, RD, MS, *Physician and Medical Director, UltraWellness Center*

"In a sometimes confusing health-information landscape, I appreciate Doc Koz's thorough approach in *Get the Func Out*— it provides an easy-to-understand roadmap to not only what could be going on, but the best first steps to take in the detoxing process. He has created a powerful tool to help support your health."

—GABBY REECE, *American Professional Volleyball Player, Sports Announcer, Model, and Host of The Gabby Reece Show*

PRAISE FOR GET THE FUNC OUT

"We normally have a wake-up call at some point where something happens—something as simple as too much stomach acid—that sets us on the journey down the rabbit hole searching for potential ways to fix our digestive issues. Everything Dr. Koz offers people to consider about nutrition and seeing things holistically is so valuable. As a huge fan of his first book, *Unfunc Your Gut,* I've told all my listeners Dr. Koz's work is an 'absolute must' for all who have food sensitivities and/or a history of gut issues, as I do. I'm so grateful for his recommended lifestyle and diet changes that probe beneath symptoms to find the root cause. After taking on the Pandora's box of gut issues, he now follows suit for hormones and detox in *Get the Func Out*—and his passion for helping people shines through."

—BRIAN KEANE, *Personal Trainer, Sports Nutritionist, Podcaster and Author of* The Fitness Mindset

"Doc Koz has done it again! In a stressed world burdened with health confusion, *Get the Func Out* provides a comprehensive yet incredibly approachable guide to tackling our toxic burden and reclaiming hormonal health. Filled with just the right blend of scientific insight, encouragement, and practical action steps, this book has become a go-to resource for my audience on their wellness journeys."

—MELANIE AVALON, *Author of* What When Wine, *and Host of* The Melanie Avalon Biohacking Podcast *and* The Intermittent Fasting Podcast

GET THE

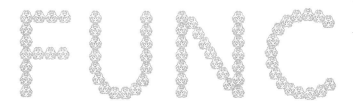

OUT

A Functional Medicine Guide
to Balance Your Hormones
and Detox

PETER KOZLOWSKI, MD

Library of Congress Cataloging-in-Publication Data

Kozlowski, Peter
Get the Func Out: A Functional Medicine Guide
to Balance Your Hormones and Detox

p. cm.
Paperback ISBN: 978-1-947708-15-0 · Ebook ISBN: 978-1-947708-28-0
Library of Congress Control Number: 2022918350
First Edition, October 2022

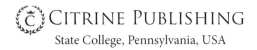

CITRINE PUBLISHING
State College, Pennsylvania, USA
(828) 585-7030 · www.CitrinePublishing.com

*Dedicated to our baby boy Carl,
the hungriest bulldog you ever met.
He was always next to me snorting
or snoring when writing this book.*

*We lost him suddenly, tragically,
and too young, but are forever grateful
for every moment with him.*

*And an even bigger dedication
to my wife, Mackenzie,
and our other bulldog, Gus,
for helping me to not give up.*

CONTENTS

INTRODUCTION

I am excited to share with you two of my favorite topics: hormones and toxins. Hormones *and* toxins? These may seem like random subjects to discuss together but rest assured, I am going to explain how they are connected. As a Family Practice doctor, I was taught how to identify which medications will help you feel better; as a Functional Medicine doctor, I was taught to be a detective for your health. I don't try to figure out how to make you feel better; I try to determine what is contributing to your illness, and through helping your body come into balance, you'll feel better. In Functional Medicine, there are five main areas where we look for imbalances; food, gut health, hormone imbalances, toxins, and mental, emotional, and spiritual health. In my first book, *Unfunc your Gut,* I introduced food, gut health, and mental, emotional, and spiritual health, which seemed unrelated but are undeniably connected. Here you'll learn the same thing about hormones and toxins.

Before we get into it, there are two important points I would like to make. First is that the following chapters come from my perspective as a clinician. While entire books have been written about each of these subjects that I dedicated only a chapter to, I am providing you the highest-yield tips and explanations that can make an impact for *how you feel.* You can get much deeper dives on many of these subjects from authors who write from the vantage points of scientists, especially those whose focus is in the laboratory. And these books can definitely help you on your journey, yet they can be complex and difficult to understand. There are also great books written from patients' viewpoints, in the words of people who actually lived with these conditions. While I am a scientist by training, my patients taught me how to apply that science to the real world, so that's what I share with you here.

The other point is that *it is very rarely as simple as "one cause for one disease."* This seems to be the focus in regular medicine, where salt equals high blood pressure and tobacco equals cancer, or from a functional medicine standpoint, where food sensitivity equals lupus, SIBO equals eczema, low testosterone equals depression, mold exposure equals neuropathy, and trauma equals anxiety. Throughout my decade plus of functional medicine experience, I've learned that *it is not one cause but it is a combination of factors that contribute to disease.* For example, food sensitivities, dysbiosis, estrogen dominance, mold toxicity and trauma equate to autoimmune disease or neurological disorders or other chronic diseases. As I teach my patients, we all have a "bucket" and if we fill that bucket with different toxic substances, it eventually overflows into disease. Rarely has our bucket overflowed due to one thing. In the doctor-patient relationship, our job is to identify what is in your bucket, empty it, and replenish it with nutrients. So let's now get into how hormones and toxins can affect your bucket.

Over 50 hormones have been identified in the human body, but don't worry, we're not going to talk about all of them here. As my patients know, I like to keep things simple.

First of all, what are hormones?

Hormones are chemical messengers that are secreted directly into the blood, which once in the blood travel to organs and tissues all over the body to do their jobs.

What are some of the jobs of hormones?

Development and growth, metabolism of food items, sexual function and reproductive health, cognitive function and mood, and maintenance of body temperature and thirst.

What are some of the most important hormone-secreting organs and what hormones do they secrete?

- **Pituitary gland:** Growth hormone (GH), thyroid stimulating hormone (TSH), follicle-stimulating hormone (FSH), adrenocorticotropic hormone (ACTH), melanocyte-stimulating hormone (MSH), luteinizing hormone (LH), prolactin, oxytocin, and vasopressin

- **Pineal Gland:** Melatonin

- **Thymus:** Thymopoietin

- **Thyroid and Parathyroid:** T4, T3, parathyroid hormone (PTH), calcitonin

- **Stomach:** Gastrin, gherkin, histamine, somatostatin, neuropeptide

- **Pancreas:** Insulin, glucagon, somatostatin

- **Liver:** Insulin-like growth factor (IGF), thrombopoietin

- **Adrenal Glands:** Androgens, glucocorticoids, adrenaline, noradrenaline

- **Kidney:** Calcitriol, renin, erythropoietin

- **Ovaries and Placenta:** Estrogens, progesterone

- **Uterus:** Prolactin, relaxin

- **Testes:** Androgens, estradiol, inhibin

Without going into unnecessary depth on all of these, we'll focus on the seven hormone imbalances I've found to be the most common and impactful: the pituitary hormones, adrenal hormones, thyroid hormones, insulin, estrogen, progesterone, and testosterone. Most probably have or have had an issue with at least one if not all of these, so we are going to learn more about how they work, how they can be damaged, how you test, and how you can improve your hormone function.

Following your learning about hormones, we're also going to talk about toxins. What are toxins? Toxins are poisonous substances which can cause disease when introduced into the body, and if they accumulate can lead to serious conditions, injury and/or death. Where do they come from? They can come from living organisms like bacteria or fungi (endotoxins) or they can be introduced into our environment (exotoxins). What are some common sources of toxins we are exposed too regularly?

- LPS from dysbiotic bacteria or yeast like candida (come from inside your body)

- Infectious diseases like viruses

- Mental, emotional, spiritual health (e.g., trauma, stress, anxiety, loneliness, etc.)

- Mycotoxins from mold in water-damaged buildings

- Heavy metals like lead, arsenic, cadmium mercury, cesium, thallium from things like air pollution, food, house dust, soil and water, cigarette smoke, groundwater, etc.

- Electromagnetic fields (EMF) from electronic equipment like cellphones and Wi-Fi

- Phthalates and parabens added to plastics to make them more flexible, found in plastic wrap for food, plastic containers, furniture, toys, shampoo, cosmetics, deodorant, perfumes, etc.

- Glyphosate sprayed on genetically modified crops like soy, corn, canola, cotton, sugar beets, alfalfa, etc.

- DDE/DDT organochlorines found in meat, poultry, dairy, and fish

- Bisphenol A (BPA) in food and beverage containers, sales receipts, water bottles, plastic dinnerware, and baby bottles

- Organophosphates found in crops, trees, lawn treatment, insect control, and livestock

- Triclosan in many personal care products: deodorants, soaps, toothpastes, shampoos, etc; kitchen utensils, toys and medical devices

- Polybrominated diphenyl ethers (PBDE) used as flame retardants in furniture, found in fish and in highest concentrations in indoor dust

- Polychlorinated biphenyls (PCBs) like dioxin found in food and some water

- Dry-cleaning chemicals

- Volatile solvents like benzene, styrene, toluene from gasoline, cigarette smoke, air fresheners, glues, paints, memory foam mattresses

- Perflourocarbons used for waterproofing, flameproofing and other protective coatings for a variety of clothes, furniture and other household items

- Benzophenone-3 in sunscreen

- Trihalomethanes from chlorinated water, showering, washing dishes, and clothes

Just to name a few…

When does your exposure to these start? Before you are even born, most can cross the placenta and many are found in breast milk. One estimate says that there are more than 1,400 chemicals[1] in our environment that are known or likely carcinogens (carcinogen means cancer causing). Another study by the Campaign for Safe Cosmetics reported that women expose themselves to over 100 individual chemicals each day through personal care products.[2] In the Halifax project, 74 scientists from 28 countries focused on the possibility that mixtures of commonly encountered chemicals in the environment may be capable of carcinogenic effects. The scientists selected 85 chemicals that were not considered to be carcinogenic to humans. The group found that 50 of those chemicals support key cancer-related mechanisms at environmentally relevant levels of exposure.[3] Simply, that means they found 50 chemicals we are exposed to regularly that fill your bucket, which when mixed together can cause cancer. That might be OK if we were just exposed to toxins, but we also fill our bucket with trauma, foods that are genetically modified, medications, processed foods, high doses of sugar, imbalanced gut bacteria, combined with tobacco and alcohol, and a lack of nutrition and sleep, with too much stress. Now you can see how our buckets can overflow. Scientifically your bucket is called your total toxic body burden.[4]

What symptoms could someone with an elevated total toxic burden (a full bucket) have?

- Fatigue
- Muscle aches
- Joint pain
- Sinus congestion
- Postnasal drip
- Headaches
- Gas/bloating
- Constipation
- Diarrhea
- Foul-smelling stools
- Heartburn
- Hormonal imbalances
- Insomnia
- Difficulty concentrating
- Food cravings
- Water retention

- Trouble losing weight
- Rashes
- Skin problems
- Eczema
- Psoriasis

- Acne
- Canker sores
- Dark circles under the eyes
- Premenstrual syndrome
- Bad breath

Under what kinds of conditions should people be considered to have elevated toxic burden?

- Progressive immune dysfunction
- Chronic infections
- Autoimmune diseases
- Endocrine problems: thyroid, adrenal, male/female hormones
- History of chemical exposure during times of high stress

- Multiple chemical sensitivities
- Infertility
- Adverse reactions of medications
- Allergies or asthma
- History of obvious industrial or agricultural exposure
- Poor caffeine tolerance

As you can see, toxins can pose a major problem to our bodies. We are exposed to an exorbitant amount of them and they can be very damaging to our organs and tissues. We will get into specific toxins and how to deal with them, but first…

How are toxins connected to hormones?

Toxins cause disruption at the cellular level at any point during the hormonal process, from the gland that produces the hormone to the tissue that receives it and many points in between.[5] And there are over 800 chemicals that are suspected to be hormone disruptors and they have been found in the blood, urine and breast milk. They accumulate over time through consistent exposure to tiny amounts (filling your bucket). Let's look at a few specific toxins which are known endocrine disruptors.

- Bisphenol A (BPA) has been found to have an affinity for estrogen receptors. This means BPA binds where your estrogen should be binding and prevents estrogen from working.[6] Studies have also found elevated rates of diabetes,[7] mammary and prostate cancers, decreased sperm count,[8] reproductive problems, early puberty,[9] obesity, and neurological problems due to elevated levels of BPA.

- Phthalates have also been found to affect estrogen but they can have pro-estrogen effects, or enhance the activity of estrogen.[10]

- Atrazine used to reduce the growth of leaves and weeds in wheat, soy, and sugar cane crops has been found to demasculinize and feminize male vertebrates.[11] That means it shrinks testicles, reduces sperm count, and can even make males grow ovaries…

- Polychlorinated bisphenols (PCBs) damage both thyroid and have estrogenic and anti-androgenic activity.[12] PCBs were banned in 1979 for their persistent pollutant effects.

- Dichlorodiphenyltrichloroethane (DDT) used as pesticides has been found to have many negative hormonal effects. It may inhibit the proper development of female reproductive organs,[13] which adversely affects reproduction into maturity. Additional studies suggest that a marked decrease in fertility in adult males may be due to DDT exposure.[14] Exposure to DDT in utero can also increase a child's risk of childhood obesity.[15]

- We will talk about many heavy metals later on, but to start with one, let's look at lead. Lead accumulates in granulosa cells of the ovary, causing delays in growth and pubertal development and reduced fertility in females. It also damages the adrenal glands as well as the thyroid.[16]

All of the above are toxins that we are being exposed too regularly. I am going to use the example of my wife Mackenzie's morning routine, to exemplify the amount of toxins a woman can be exposed to just going through a regular morning routine (the following is not 100% her typical day, but it is close and could be for you or someone you know).

Thinking holistically, let's start "the morning" with when and how she goes to bed. And let's say we didn't know the dangers of memory foam mattresses. Memory foam mattresses are made from polyurethane foam mixed with petrol chemicals (to make it "memory foam") and flame retardants (PBDE). Each mattress can be a little different, since different companies have different secret recipes; however, one study found 61 petroleum-based compounds in a single mattress.[17] These are otherwise known as volatile organic compounds (VOC), which have been found to change the excretion of hormones in urine.[18] And say she sleeps with her smart phone on the nightstand (she doesn't) and the wireless router in the next room. Not to mention our house is located next to large power lines and a brand-new cell phone tower around the corner (fortunately, it isn't). These are creating electromagnetic (EMF) fields, which are streams of invisible energy waves that can add to our bucket. According to the World Health Organization (WHO), EMFs are possibly carcinogenic to humans. Three different studies found anywhere between 1.4 to 2 times increased risk of leukemia in children from EMF exposure.[19,20,21] Another study suggested that long-term exposure to EMF may lead to depression, stress, anxiety, and poor sleep quality.[22]

Mackenzie's bucket is filling up just by sleeping (which really stinks because sleep is when our body is recovering and healing),

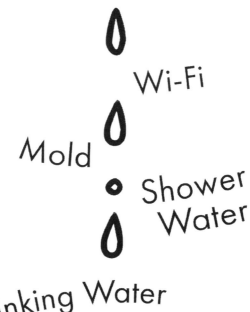

Wi-Fi

Mold

Shower
Water

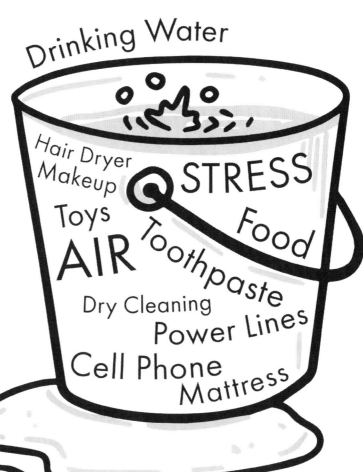

Drinking Water

Hair Dryer
Makeup

STRESS

Toys

Food

AIR Toothpaste

Dry Cleaning

Power Lines

Cell Phone

Mattress

but I have more bad news: our house had water damage two years ago and we had a mold problem (fortunately, in reality it doesn't). But in our hypothetical example, we hired some local remediator and they said they problem was gone. However, the first thing that I learned in Environmental Medicine is that the only treatment for a moldy house is to knock it down. This is debatable, but if our remediation didn't work and Mackenzie is breathing in mycotoxins like ochratoxin A from Aspergillus mold and Verrucarin A from Stachybotrys mold while she's sleeping, her bucket is getting even fuller. We are going to dive deep into mold in Chapter 8 as it is one of the most common toxins I work with, but for now let's just say that various studies have found various detrimental effects of mold, including neurologic, respiratory,[23] and immune disorders.[24]

Mackenzie hasn't even gotten out of bed yet and she's already added quite bit to her toxin burden. When she does get up, she starts her day with a shot of glutathione (she actually does this, as it's the body's master antioxidant—more to come in Chapter 6; this started when she was detoxing from mold, so she actually supports her detox ability). Next she has a glass of water straight out of the faucet. There have been more toxins found in the first world's drinking water than I could name, but a few include lead (from lead pipes and plumbing fixtures), atrazine (from pesticides), pathogens (bacteria, viruses, parasites), chlorine treatment byproducts (like trihalomethane and halo acetic acids), arsenic (enters our water from industrial and agricultural pollution), nitrates (from fertilizers), vinyl chloride (used to make PVC plastic products), and pharmaceuticals. (*What?!?* Yes, prescription drugs enter our water when people taking them pee out the metabolites and flush them.) Yikes.

After having water, she checks her phone and sees the breaking news from the past day and checks in on her favorite social media apps. This activates her stress response, which has been shown to negatively affect enzymes that help break down fat and detox prescription drugs.[25] She then heads to her workout, where again she is supporting detox. Toxins are fat soluble; detox is when our body makes them water soluble and then we get rid of them through our urine, stool, and sweat (much more to come on this in Chapter 6). So a great way to detox is sweating! Not to mention a good morning poop. Another win for Mackenzie. At least she has a couple things in her morning routine that help detox.

Breakfast is next and breakfast six days a week is a smoothie. The recipe can vary, but let's say there are strawberries, blueberries, banana, and spinach. Unfortunately, strawberries and spinach are numbers 1 and 2 on the Environmental Working Group's (EWG) Dirty Dozen; blueberries are number 16 and bananas are number 28. The Dirty Dozen is a catalog of conventionally grown fruits and vegetables with the highest amount of pesticides. When you look into the Dirty Dozen it is pretty scary:

> "More than 90 percent of samples of strawberries, apples, cherries, spinach, nectarines, and leafy greens tested positive for residues of two or more pesticides. A single sample of kale, collard and mustard greens had up to 20 different pesticides. On average, spinach samples had 1.8 times as much pesticide residue by weight as any other crop tested." [26]

Just an FYI: the EWG also publishes the Clean Fifteen, which is a catalog of conventionally grown fruits and vegetables with the lowest amount of pesticides. Both these lists are updated yearly; the top five cleanest in 2021 were avocados, sweet corn, pineapple, onions, and papaya. Let's get back to breakfast. Mackenzie also puts a protein powder in her smoothie, even though researchers for the Clean Label Project screened 134 protein powders for 130 types of toxins and found that many protein powders contained heavy metals (lead, arsenic, cadmium, and mercury), bisphenol-A (BPA, which is used to make plastic), pesticides, or other contaminants with links to cancer and other health conditions.[27] She then blends her smoothie using almond milk she got at the grocery store; one study showed that store-bought almond milk might only be made of 2% almonds, while the rest is water with emulsifiers, possibly sweetener, along with nutrients such as vitamin A and D that have been artificially added. When she was making that smoothie, in her head it was a healthy breakfast.

Since the smoothie is frozen and the mornings in the mountains in Montana can be chilly, sometimes she drinks the smoothie while taking a hot shower. Similar to drinking water, shower water comes from the same source and can contain chemicals such as chlorine, disinfection byproducts (DBPs), volatile organic compounds (VOCs), fluoride, fluoride, pharmaceuticals, heavy metals, and nitrates. And the water her skin absorbs from the shower might actually be worse than the morning cup of water, not to mention the steam she breathes.

Did you know it's actually pretty easy to make almond milk? Here is a recipe from my good friend Jonny Juicer.

Jonny Juicer's Almond Milk
— 1 cup of soaked almonds (6 hours)
— 3 cups of water
— 1 teaspoon of Vanilla Extract
— 3 pitted dates (for sweetness)

Blend all of the ingredients and strain in a nut bag. This should provide roughly 1 liter of almond milk. Enjoy!

According to a recent study, 50 to 80 percent of dissolved chemicals in water are released into the air when water is heated.[28] So when we shower in hot water, those chemicals are released into the air and we breathe them in throughout the duration of our showers.

Next Mackenzie brushes her teeth. Did you know toothpaste can contain ingredients such as triclosan, propylene glycol, detergent, thickening and flavoring agents, and artificial sweeteners, all of which could be problematic for your health?[29] After brushing, she breaks out the hair dryer, having no idea that a hair dryer can actually emit more EMFs than her cell phone. EMFs are measured in mG (milliGauss). When a phone is ringing, the maximum levels range between 9-15 mG, while an average blow-dryer's EMF level is between 35 to 100 mG (milliGauss). There are low-EMF hair dryers out there and if you are using one that you are not sure about and have symptoms like compromised immune system, headaches, chronic fatigue, irritability, poor sleep, hormonal disorders, or brain fog you may want to invest in a new hair dryer. A new hair dryer will not solve all your health issues, but the best way I describe Functional Medicine is that we are emptying your bucket. So the more things we take out of your bucket, the better your chances for healing are.

After her hair is dry, she straightens it using a hair straightener and that is really good because formaldehyde has been used in many hair-straightening products.[30] The next step to get ready for the day is makeup. Mackenzie is naturally very beautiful and doesn't need much. In 2013, researchers at the University of Berkely tested 32 different lipsticks and lip glosses commonly found in drugstores and department stores. They detected lead, cadmium, chromium, aluminum and five other metals in different lipsticks.[31] Per- and polyfluoroalkyl substances (PFAS) are a class of chemicals, which includes PFOA, PFOS, and GenX. These chemicals can bioaccumulate in bodies over time and have been linked to cancer, thyroid disease, liver damage, decreased fertility, and hormone disruption. PFAS substances were found in 52% of 231 makeup products purchased in the United States and Canada. Some of the highest levels were found in foundations (63%), waterproof mascara (82%), and long-lasting lipstick (62%), according to a study published in the journal *Environmental Science & Technology Letters.* And as if anything could possibly be worse, the study found some 88% of the tested products failed to disclose on their labels any ingredients that would explain those chemical markers, even though that is a requirement of the US Food and Drug Administration.[32]

Next Mackenzie gets dressed and is now ready to head out to start her day. But since I just took her clothes to the dry cleaner, we run into another problem, tetrachloroethylenel (a.k.a. perchloroethylene, or perc) is the predominant solvent used for dry cleaning.[33] Why is that bad? Perc has cancer-causing and toxic effects on the central nervous system, kidneys, liver, respiratory system, eyes and skin, and on reproduction and development.

Before she walks out the door, there is still the most important part of her morning routine—play with our bulldogs Gus and Carl. It's really nice: she steps into the yard and breathes the air that you would think is fresh but according to the EPA, it contains carbon monoxide, lead, nitrogen dioxide, ozone, particulate matter of different size fractions, and sulfur dioxide.[34] These six different toxins found in our air regularly. Gus and Carl don't care so they bring her their favorite dog toys full of polyvinyl chloride (PVC), phthalates, bisphenol A (BPA), lead, chromium, formaldehyde, cadmium, and bromine.[35] These are the toxins commonly found in pet products. Another good thing that we started was cutting out dog food for Gus and Carl. We cook for them twice a week, as dog food has been found to be full of mold mycotoxins.[36]

Again, yikes, that is a lot of toxic burden to place on your body, doing what we consider 'normal' routine things. What is even worse is that you typically don't smell, taste or feel these chemicals, so you have no idea it's happening. And when you go to a traditional doctor, they run their normal tests that come back saying "everything is great and normal," but you return home knowing deep down that *not everything is normal.* That's why I am so excited to dive into these topics deeper and give you a huge head start on your healing journey.

CHAPTER 1

The Thyroid

We are going to get things kicked off with the thyroid. Why the thyroid? According to the American Thyroid Association, more than 12% of people in the United States will develop a thyroid disease, but about 60% of those with thyroid disease are unaware. An estimated 20 million Americans have some form of thyroid disease. Women are 5 to 8 times more likely to have thyroid issues.[37] So we are going to start with the thyroid because thyroid disease is extremely common. In fact, if you have an issue with your thyroid, more than likely you don't know it.

The thyroid gland sits in your neck just below your Adam's apple. It is made up of two lobes, which rest on both sides of your windpipe, each about the size of a plum cut in half, joined in the middle by the isthmus. It makes two hormones that are secreted into the blood: thyroxine (T4) and triiodothyronine (T3). Most of the tissues in your body have thyroid receptors. These hormones are necessary for just about all the cells in your body to work normally. T4 derived its name because it contains four atoms of iodine, while T3 has three.

In the cells and tissues of the body, the T4 is converted to T3. T3 that is directly made by the gland, or T3 that is converted from T4, is the biologically active hormone, which interacts with cells and tissues all over your body.

T3 influences the *metabolism*, the speed with which your body cells work. Your skin and hair growth are dependent on T3, which functions like a growth hormone for your skin and hair cells. If you don't produce enough thyroid hormone, the growth cycle of the skin and hair (which are very rapid) gets broken and the outer layers of your skin can be damaged and become dry, your skin can turn yellow, your hair can fall out or become coarse and brittle, and your fingernails can get weak.

T3 influences how strongly your heart pumps and how quickly it beats. Not enough thyroid hormone can slow your heart rate, while too much can make you have palpitations. T3 also influences the elasticity of your blood vessels; if there is not enough thyroid hormone, your blood vessels become more elastic and your blood pressure must increase in order to carry oxygen and nutrients to your tissues.

Normal function of your muscles is dependent on sufficient thyroid hormone. Therefore, if your thyroid hormone production is low you can feel muscle weakness and pain (this is what is meant when people say "low thyroid"). This goes for your gut as well. Low thyroid can cause low stomach acid, poor absorption, constipation, gallstones, and overgrowths or imbalances in your microbiome.

As you can see, the thyroid is pretty important! But you may be wondering if I have any clue what I'm talking about because I haven't even mentioned Thyroid Stimulating Hormone (TSH) and for many of you that is probably the only hormone that your doctor mentioned and tested when you asked whether your thyroid wasn't working properly.

Let me give you an analogy of how the thyroid works. Think of it like the heating system in your home. When you set the temperature to 70 degrees Fahrenheit in your home, the thermostat monitors the temperature; when the thermostat detects that the temperature drops below 70 degrees (which happens frequently during the winter in my hometown of Bozeman, Montana), it sends a signal to the heater to produce more heat. When the temperature is back to 70 degrees, the signal turns off, and the heater turns off.

In your body, your pituitary gland is your thermostat, the signal it releases is TSH, and your thyroid is your heater; the heat it produces is T4 and T3. If your heat was not working properly, would you want your heating repair person to only check your thermostat or would you want them to check your heater as well? I would want them to check both! I have racked my brain trying to remember when I was taught in medical school and residency to test only TSH to assess someone's thyroid function and what was the reason for this. I cannot remember. I have no clue honestly, I can't make sense of it. When I started training in Functional Medicine, I was taught to test all three: TSH, free T4, and free T3 (free means circulating hormone that is not bound to protein and is able to attach to receptors), and luckily this has been all I've done my whole career. I cannot tell you how many patients I have met with a normal TSH but a low T4 or T3. Or an elevated TSH but a normal T4 or T3 level. The patient with a low T4 or T3, I would treat for low thyroid, whereas someone with normal T4 and T3 levels despite an elevated TSH, I would not treat, but I would continue to test that person every 3 to 6 months, as the thyroid can change.

The top ten symptoms that would make me test someone's thyroid are:

- Fatigue
- Constipation
- Depression
- Weight gain
- Cold hands and feet
- Dry hair and skin
- Hair loss
- Menstrual irregularities
- Edema (swelling of your extremities)
- Muscle aches and/or joint pain

If someone's thyroid came back looking abnormal, I would then also order other tests to try to identify the source of dysfunction. First would be two different thyroid antibodies: Thyroid peroxidase antibodies (TPO) and Anti-Thyroglobulin antibodies (Tg). Measuring levels of thyroid antibodies can help diagnose an autoimmune thyroid disorder such as Graves' disease (the most common cause of hyperthyroidism) and (Hashimoto's disease) the most common cause of hypothyroidism. Thyroid antibodies are made when your immune system gets confused, recognizes your thyroid as an invader, wants to get rid of it, and so it attacks the thyroid gland by mistake. Why would this happen? The best analogy I have heard about the thyroid that I learned from Dr. Susan Blum, one of my mentors, is that the thyroid is a like a sponge for toxins. What else are we talking about in this book? Toxins. Again you see the connection. When your thyroid absorbs consistent amounts of heavy metals, mycotoxins, glyphosate, and endotoxins from imbalanced bacteria, just to name a few, it could make your immune system think the thyroid is the problem and want to eliminate it.

There are some imaging studies that can be ordered as well, the most common being an ultrasound of the thyroid. The ultrasound can help you identify thyroid nodules, which are little lumps made of abnormal growths of thyroid cells. Sometimes your doctor may be able to feel them without the ultrasound. Surprisingly, thyroid nodules are not something to worry about generally; by age 60, about one-half of all people have a thyroid nodule. It's important to know that about 95% of such nodules are benign (non-cancerous).[38] Their cause is not clear, though they are more commonly found in patients diagnosed with Hashimoto's or iodine deficiency. Is it possible the thyroid cells are growing abnormally into nodules due to all the toxins that we are being exposed to everyday? It wouldn't shock me. If you do have nodules, your doctor may order a Fine Needle

Aspiration, which is a way to see whether or not the cells are cancerous. If you have been diagnosed with an overactive thyroid that is producing too much hormone, then your doctor may do a Radioactive Iodine Uptake Test to try to understand why you are producing too much thyroid hormone.

In my practice, I would also want to look at some of your vitamins and nutrients. Your thyroid needs vitamins and minerals to function properly. Some of the most important ones are iodine, selenium, zinc, iron, vitamin A, and vitamin D.[39,40] Some of these can be difficult to test so if someone has thyroid issues, we may start them on these supplements to support the thyroid.

Nutrient	Function	Test	Supplementation to consider
Iodine	Needed for T4 and T3 production	Urinary fasting morning spot	150 mcg per day. Only take if your iodine levels are low and your doctor prescribes. Too much iodine can be a big problem for proper thyroid function. It is over prescribed in the alternative medicine world, personally I very rarely use it.
Selenium	Needed for T4 and T3 production, also protects thyroid from oxidative damage (toxins)	RBC selenium levels	200-400 mcg per day
Zinc	Needed for T4 and T3 production	RBC zinc levels	15-30mg per day
Iron	Needed for proper conversion of T4 to T3	CBC and ferritin (the amount of iron stored in your body)	15-20mg – Only take if your iron levels are low and your doctor prescribes

Nutrient	Function	Test	Supplementation to consider
Vitamin A	Has been shown to regulate thyroid hormone metab-olism and inhibit thyroid-stimu-lating hormone (TSH) secretion[41]	Serum vitamin A (rarely ordered)	10,000 iu per day or 900 mcg for men and 700mcg for women; only take if prescribed by your doctor
Vitamin D	Regulates gene expression and modulates immune system; deficiency found in both Hashimoto's and Graves' disease[42]	Vitamin D 25 OH blood test	Dose based on your levels, can range between 2,000-10,000k iu per day or more; too much vitamin D can be toxic

There are also some Functional Medicine tests that I would like to do.

Condition	Test	Why?	Instructions
Low Stomach Acid	Baking Soda Test or Betaine HCl supplementation	If you're not digesting, you're not absorbing your nutrients, even if your diet is "healthy." Your thyroid needs nutrients! See page 5.	Found in *Unfunc Your Gut*
Food Sensitivities	Elimination diet	Can create toxins which are absorbed by thy-roid; gluten could possibly block your thyroid[43]	Found in *Unfunc Your Gut*
Dysbiosis & SIBO	Stool, urine, breath testing	Can create toxins which are absorbed by thyroid	Found in *Unfunc Your Gut*, ordered by your Func-tional Medicine doctor.

Condition	Test	Why?	Instructions
Toxins	Urine	Toxins can be absorbed by the thyroid	Details coming soon! Keep reading. Ordered by your Functional Medicine doctor.
Stress	Listening to the patient's story	Stress appears to play an important role in autoimmune thyroid disease through activation of neuroendocrine pathways[44]	If you have read *Unfunc Your Gut*, you know mental, emotional, and spiritual health is my passion and should always be the most important thing we are working on for our health.

Also make sure you are not taking something which is blocking your thyroid. Medications that can block thyroid production or function include:

- Betablockers
- Birth control
- Estrogen replacement
- Lithium
- Phenytoin
- Theophylline
- Chemotherapy
- And others

We obviously want to order the basic tests as well.

Test	Reference Range	Optimal
TSH	0.40- 4.5 mIU/L	0.40 – 2.5 mIU/L
Free T4	0.8-1.8 ng/dl	1 – 1.5 ng/dl
Free T3	2.3-4.2 pg/ml	3.2 – 4.5 pg/ml
TPO	<9 IU/ml	arguably 0
Thyroglobulin Antibodies	< or = 1 IU/ml	arguably 0
Reverse T3*	11-31 ng/dl	11-18 ng/dl

The difference between me as a Functional Medicine doctor and a family practice doctor is that if I were a traditional doc, I would probably only order a TSH level and treat your thyroid if it is too low or too high. As a Functional Medicine physician, I would order all these numbers and help you optimize your thyroid depending on what we found.

*A note on reverse T3 (rT3): I personally do not find it useful and do not test for it, however there are a number of practitioners in my field that do like to test it. The body can convert T4 into rT3, an inactive form of T3 that is incapable of the metabolic activity that is normally carried out by T3. It is believed that the body produces rT3 in times of severe illness or starvation as a mechanism for preserving energy. From a Functional Medicine perspective, my opinion is that it is produced due to toxin burden on the thyroid. I only like to order labs that are going to change my treatment plan, and reverse T3 doesn't change anything for me. I will be looking for toxins and imbalances regardless of rT3 levels.

So what are your options if you have been diagnosed with thyroid dysfunction? There are many! It is much more likely to be diagnosed with Hashimoto's (5 in 100 people)[45] than Graves' disease, (1 in 200 people).[46]

Hashimoto's and Graves' are similar as they are both considered autoimmune conditions, but Hashimoto's causes you to stop making thyroid hormone and Graves' causes you to make too much thyroid hormone. Hashimoto's would typically present as a high TSH, and low T4 and/or T3; you may also have positive TPO or thyroglobulin antibodies. Whereas Graves' would present as low TSH and high T4 and/or T3, with possibly positive antibodies as well.

My experience is much greater in working with hypothyroidism than hyper. There are many patients I have worked with who have low thyroid hormone without antibodies, so that is not Hashimoto's, but is still treated as low thyroid.

Labs	RX plan
High TSH, normal T4 and T3	Do Functional Medicine testing for underlying sources of inflammation.
High TSH, normal T4, low T3.	Supplements listed above to support T4 conversion to T3. Consider T3 replacement. Do Functional Medicine testing for underlying sources of inflammation.
High TSH, low T4 and T3	Supplements listed above T4 or T3 replacement, or combo T4/T3 replacement.
Low TSH, High T4 and/or T3	Referral to Endocrinology. Do Functional Medicine testing for underlying sources of inflammation.
If thyroid is low or high, will test for Thyroid antibodies	If positive, Ultrasound, FNA (if nodules), and Radioactive Iodine Uptake Test (if high thyroid positive antibodies, consider Low-Dose Naltrexone (LDN) under your doctor's prescription.

Remember, this is just an outline. In Functional Medicine, we always individualize care. This chart is simply meant to help you understand your labs and what possible options could be. Always work with your doctor to make a plan that fits you.

Another area of significant disagreement that you might encounter from your traditional doctor is using anything other than Levothyroxine (T4 replacement sold under the brand name Synthroid), for thyroid hormone replacement, when there are more options. These are the medicines that I would consider for replacing thyroid hormone:

Thyroid Replacement Type	Generic Name	Brand Name
T4 Hormone	Levothyroxine	Synthroid
T3 Hormone	Liothyronine	Cytomel
T4/T3 combo	Desiccated porcine thyroid 4 parts T4 1 part T3	Armour Nature-throid
T4/T3 combo	Compounded to your levels	Made specific to you by a compounding pharmacy

I have had success with all of these options, so how do we decide which one is the best for you? Your regular doctor would say Synthroid, your alternative medicine doc would say Armour, and I would say I don't know—the only way to find out is to try. I have had many patients come to me begging for Armour because they have read that it is better than the Synthroid their doc is giving them. There are even a few studies that suggested not all patients are satisfied with T4 replacement medications.[47,48,49] In many cases I have seen that to be true, but not for everyone. It is a trial-and-error process in my experience. If someone comes to me on Synthroid and their labs look optimal but they don't feel optimal, I will try a switch to a "desiccated thyroid" (the generic name for a medication that is 4 parts T4 1 part T3), but we may end up switching back again. If their T4 is normal but T3 is low, I might add Cytomel. We keep trying until we find what is optimal for that person.

Ultimately, you want to optimize your thyroid levels without suppressing TSH totally. Cardiovascular disease, dysrhythmias, and fractures were increased in patients with a "high TSH" and "suppressed TSH" when compared to patients with a TSH in the laboratory reference range.[50] Patients with a "low TSH" did not have an increased risk of any of these outcomes. T3 administered to older individuals may cause adverse cardiac events; excessive T3 can lead to suppression of TSH and therefore a host of side effects including cardiovascular risk and osteoporosis. Symptoms to watch out for that could present if you are taking too much thyroid hormone or medication:

- Weight loss
- Tremor
- Headache
- Upset stomach
- Vomiting
- Diarrhea
- Stomach cramps
- Nervousness
- Rapid heartbeat
- Irritability
- Insomnia
- Excessive sweating
- Increased appetite
- Fever
- Changes in menstrual cycle
- Sensitivity to heat
- Temporary hair loss

Why will your regular doctor not consider desiccated thyroid? I am not sure. Desiccated thyroid contains all four natural thyroid hormones: iodine, thyroglobulin, protein, and glandular tissue and some studies suggest it works better.[51,52] Desiccated thyroid medications have been used since 1892 and were approved by the Food and Drug Administration in 1939. Levothyroxine has been used since 1949 and liothyronine after that. Both natural and synthetic versions are approved by the FDA and made to reference standards approved by the USP. But the argument by traditional doctors is that you can't rely on the dose being accurate for desiccated hormones, and there is some truth to that. NP thyroid (desiccated) was recalled in April 2021 and September 2020 for sub-potency; Nature-thyroid had the same issue in September 2020.[53,54] However in March 2020, levothyroxine and liothyronine were recalled as well over quality concerns.[55] My personal experience in prescribing all these options has led me to listen to my patients and make a decision based on their history.

A fantastic option that I learned through my Functional Medicine training is the use of low-dose naltrexone (LDN).

Naltrexone is a competitive opiate receptor antagonist developed in the 1970s and was FDA approved in 1984 at doses ranging from 50 to 300mg to treat opiate abuse. It is given as a long-acting injection prescribed to block the euphoric and sedative effects of an opioid drug like heroin or morphine; it is now also approved to treat alcoholism.

In 1982, a man by the name of Ian Zagon discovered that naltrexone in low doses triggers an increase in the production of naturally occurring opioid compounds (a.k.a. endorphins), which have effects on cell proliferation and healing. A New York physician named Bernard Bihari found that LDN led to improved immune function in HIV/AIDS patients. It was this work that led to experimenting with LDN in other immune disorders.

How does it work for autoimmune thyroid disease?

- LDN blocks opioid growth factor (OGF) receptors for a few hours and displaces endorphins from opioid receptors.

- Cells sense opioid deficiency, which leads them to increase endorphin production

- Increased endorphin activity results in improved modulation of the immune system.

Remember autoimmune thyroid diseases are caused by an imbalanced immune response.

So how does LDN help?[56,57,58,59,60,61,62]

- Reduces overall inflammation
- Reduce levels of anti-thyroid antibodies
- Improve thyroid transport into cells
- Increase T4 to T3 conversion
- Reduce T4 to reverse T3 conversion

Wow, sounds like a miracle drug! I have seen this to be the case in many patients. Over 75% of my Hashimoto's patients who have tried LDN have reported significant improvements in their sense of well-being. But it doesn't work for everyone. I have had patients stop treatment, though not many, due to potential side effects which include:

- Anxiety
- Nausea
- Drowsiness
- Headache
- Abdominal pain
- Insomnia
- Diarrhea
- Anorexia
- Muscle pain
- Vivid dreams (Most common)
- Mood changes
- Trouble concentrating

Case Study: Jennifer

Let's look at a patient, Jennifer, who came to see me because of her thyroid. She was a 47-year-old female who grew up in Eastern Europe and had been exposed to radiation from the Chernobyl nuclear disaster. She was diagnosed with Hashimoto's at the age of 35 and had been having issues getting it under control since that time. She came in with symptoms of fatigue, cold hands and feet, thinning hair, dry skin, bloating, constipation, gas, strong stool odor, and difficulty concentrating. She was having normal periods every 26 to 29 days. She had trauma from immigrating, a poor relationship with her husband, and spent a lot of time online reading about thyroid disease. Before seeking my care, she had seen another doctor who had ordered bloodwork just three weeks earlier. Here are her labs and a reminder of reference ranges.

Test	Jennifer's Value	Reference Range	Optimal
TSH	12.68 mIU/L	0.40- 4.5 mIU/L	0.40 – 2.5 mIU/L
Free T4	1.1 ng/dl	0.8-1.8 ng/dl	1 – 1.5 ng/dl
Free T3	3.1 ng/dl	2.3-4.2 pg/ml	3.2 – 4.5 pg/ml

Test	Jennifer's Value	Reference Range	Optimal
TPO	3219	<9 IU/ml	arguably 0
Ferritin	5.2	16-232 ng/ml	50-100 ng/ml
Vitamin D	48	30-100 ng/mL	50-80 ng/ml
Thyroid Ultrasound done 6 months earlier	One nodule found to be benign		

So we had an elevated TSH by all standards, a free T4 within reference and optimal range, a free T3 within reference range and just below optimal range, the highest elevation in thyroid antibodies I had seen to that point in my practice, low iron stores both out of reference and optimal range, and a vitamin D within reference range but just below optimal.

Jennifer came in adamant that she wanted to go on thyroid hormone replacement. Going over her lab work and symptoms, I did think a very small dose of thyroid hormone was an option, but not the best option. I explained to her all the benefits of LDN and thought this was the best way to go. Then I also recommended a Functional medicine workup, including an Elimination Diet following low FODMAP principles (aka the Koz Plan, see the recipes in *Unfunc Your Gut),* SIBO and stool testing because of her GI symptoms, with a long-term plan of looking at her toxin levels after we unfunc'ed her gut. She ended up agreeing to try LDN as she had already experimented with thyroid hormone replacement in the past. The dosing regimen we followed was:

- 1 capsule of 1.5 mg naltrexone at bedtime for 2 weeks
- 1 capsule of 3 mg naltrexone at bedtime for 2 weeks
- Then, 1 capsule of 4.5 mg naltrexone at bedtime thereafter

LDN can be made in capsules, sublingual, and creams, I have used them all. I also recommended an iron supplement (20mg daily) and vitamin D (2,000iu daily), as she was already taking selenium and zinc. Most importantly I advised her to get off the Internet, trust me, start meditating, and make her mental, emotional, and spiritual health the focus of her health. When she came back six weeks later to go over her gut results, she reported not starting the Elimination Diet and not feeling too much different, but had been taking LDN nightly. She went to the lab before her visit to check in on her thyroid and these were her results.

Test	Jennifer's Value	Reference Range	Optimal
TSH	10.01 mIU/L	0.40- 4.5 mIU/L	0.40 – 2.5 mIU/L
Free T4	1.3 ng/dl	0.8-1.8 ng/dl	1 – 1.5 ng/dl
Free T3	3.3 ng/dl	2.3-4.2 pg/ml	3.2 – 4.5 pg/ml
TPO	311	<9 IU/ml	arguably 0
Ferritin	30	16-232 ng/ml	50-100 ng/ml
Vitamin D	75	30-100 ng/mL	50-80 ng/ml

Wow! That looked great! Antibodies decreased from 3219 to 311, TSH went down from 12.68 to 10.01, free T4 increased from 1.1 to 1.3, and free T3 went up from 3.1 to 3.3, was now in optimal range. Her iron also improved and vitamin D was optimized. Her stool testing showed dysbiosis and SIBO. I kept her on LDN, prescribed a gut-healing regimen, continued iron daily and switched vitamin D to every other day since winter was coming.

Jennifer came back three months later reporting that her GI symptoms had totally resolved and her hypothyroid symptoms also all improved. She had way more energy, her hair was not thinning as much, her skin was softer, and her cold intolerance was much improved. She also said she had started couples therapy and had tried meditation. She did not follow the Elimination Diet but stayed mostly low FODMAP. She was ecstatic and so was I! And take a look at her labs 18 weeks after starting treatment:

Test	Jennifer's Value	Reference Range	Optimal
TSH	5.88 mIU/L	0.40- 4.5 mIU/L	0.40 – 2.5 mIU/L
Free T4	1.4 ng/dl	0.8-1.8 ng/dl	1 – 1.5 ng/dl
Free T3	3.4 ng/dl	2.3-4.2 pg/ml	3.2 – 4.5 pg/ml
TPO	69	<9 IU/ml	arguably 0
Ferritin	85	16-232 ng/ml	50-100 ng/ml
Vitamin D	82	30-100 ng/mL	50-80 ng/ml

Pretty amazing, right! A decrease in thyroid antibodies from 3219 to 69 in 18 weeks is hard to believe. An important note here: her TSH decreased from 12.68 to 5.88, which is still not in reference range, but in my opinion TSH is the least important number in the thyroid panel even though it is the only number most of your doctors have ever tested. Because she personally (via immigrating and relationships) and her thyroid (via radiation and toxins) had been through a lot, it was not surprising her TSH was elevated, but because her free T4 and T3 were optimal— and more importantly, she felt optimal—we kept her on her regimen with planned follow-up lab testing. The piece that put everything together was that Jennifer was working on her mental, emotional, spiritual health.

CHAPTER 2

The Adrenals

The adrenal glands have gained a lot of fame because they are known as your "**stress glands.**" Given my belief that your mental, emotional, and spiritual health is the most important dimension of your health, we will emphasize that aspect. But before we go there, the adrenal glands also have other essential functions that are important to understand.

The adrenal glands sit on top of your kidneys. You have two, one on top of each kidney. The one on the right sits close to the right lobe of your liver and the one on the left is close to your stomach, pancreas, and spleen. The adrenal glands are made up of two different parts: the medulla and the cortex, both of which make different hormones.

The cortex is divided into three different regions. Naming the different regions was a common question that was tough to remember on med school exams:

- **Zona Glomerulosa:** produces and secretes mineralocorticoids such as aldosterone.

- **Zona Fasciculata:** produces and secretes corticosteroids such as cortisol. It also secretes a small amount of androgens.

- **Zona Reticularis:** produces and secretes sex hormones known as androgens. DHEA, the main one, is a precursor to estradiol and testosterone. (But the ovaries and testes make much more estradiol and testosterone.) It also secretes a small amount of corticosteroids.

The medulla is in the center of the gland and secretes catecholamines (such as adrenaline, otherwise known as epinephrine, and noradrenaline, known as norepinephrine) into the bloodstream in response to stress. These are the hormones that produce the "fight or flight" response.

The hormones secreted from the cortex are considered to be vital to life—you can't live without them, whereas catecholamines from the medulla are nonessential to life.

Now let's get into the different hormones, how they affect your body, and imbalances that could occur. We will defer the androgen discussion until Chapters 5 and 6.

Aldosterone

Aldosterone is a mineralocorticoid whose main role is to regulate salt and water in the body, hence influencing your blood pressure. Our body has a set amount of salt it requires to have balance. When there is too much salt in the blood (from you diet), the salt draws more water to help lower the ratio of salt to water; and more water increases the volume of your blood which increases your blood pressure. This is why people with high blood pressure are told to eat a diet lower in salt.

Let's talk about salt briefly, because salt can be a toxin.

Salt has been vilified as always being bad, but it is not. We need salt to regulate blood pressure, heartbeat, metabolism, electrical activity, hydration, nerve function, hemoglobin production, and bone building. How much salt "the experts" say you should have in your diet seems to change almost every year and can be very confusing. The American Heart Association recommends a maximum of 2,300 mg of salt per day, but average Americans could eat anywhere between 4,000 to 10,000 mg per day. In my opinion, the most important issue is not how much salt we're eating, but the type of salt were eating. Table salt is what most people eat and table salt can be a toxin, because it is bleached and filled with additives, preservatives, anti-caking agents, moisture absorbents, fluoride, and dextrose. It is also stripped of natural mineral content and has an altered chemical nature.

Meanwhile real salt is natural, unrefined, full of all known minerals in trace amounts, and is a good source of potassium, magnesium, and calcium. The ideal type of salt is dried from a healthy sea (a.k.a. sea salt) but the problem is that chemical dumping, oil spills, and pollution in our water have ruined much of this salt as well. Currently I recommend using only Celtic, Himalayan, or Real Salt from Redmond, Utah. Even if you are eating good salt, I would not recommend eating 4,000 to 10,0000 mg per day; I would stick to a max of 2,300 mg. The main benefit will be that you are not adding another toxin to your bucket.

Aldosterone disorders can present if you make too much or too little aldosterone, or if your intake of salt is so high that your body cannot keep up with aldosterone production. Aldosterone disorders do not tend to be a "Functional Medicine issue" and are best evaluated by a specialist like an endocrinologist. Too much aldosterone can present as high blood pressure and low potassium (which could cause arrhythmia), and is usually due to a tumor secreting aldosterone. Too little aldosterone production can present as low blood pressure and elevated potassium, and this is usually due to a general loss of adrenal function or genetic mutations.

From a Functional Medicine perspective, to keep your aldosterone balanced, eat a maximum of 2,300 mg of a healthy salt per day and drink half your body weight in water (180 lbs = 90 oz of water per day).

Stress

Let's get into the good stuff now, your "stress" hormones. It's my favorite subject to talk about, but usually my patients' least favorite topic. Let's start with cortisol.

Cortisol is one of the two hormones you don't want too much of, the other being insulin. As with most things, a little bit of cortisol is OK, but too much can be a problem. There are cortisol receptors all over your body, as it helps with blood sugar regulation, metabolism, inflammation, memory formation, blood pressure control; and it supports a fetus during pregnancy. So chronic imbalances in your cortisol levels can cause chronic inflammatory conditions like elevated or low blood sugars and imbalanced blood pressure.

Traditional medicine acknowledges high cortisol under the label Cushing's syndrome, during which someone will display a flushed face, weight gain in their face, abdomen, and chest, high blood pressure, irregular periods, and skin issues. They also acknowledge low cortisol which is known as Addison's disease, which can present as fatigue, muscle and weight loss, mood swings, and skin changes. Cushing's could be due to chronic use of steroid medications like those prescribed for asthma, auto-immune conditions, a tumor of the adrenals or pituitary gland. Addison's disease can be caused by an autoimmune condition, injury, infection, surgery, cancer, and/or genetic issues.

Are there any other causes of imbalanced cortisol? That depends on who you ask. In Functional Medicine, we work with a condition called Adrenal Fatigue. Before you read any further, be aware that the Endocrinology Society and all the other traditional medical specialties do not recognize this condition. The endocrinologists go so far as to say that no scientific proof exists to support adrenal fatigue as a true medical condition. If you talk to a Functional Medicine doctor, they would probably say the majority of their patients are dealing with some degree of adrenal fatigue. I am going to share my experience as a traditionally trained Medical Doctor who switched to Functional Medicine. I would say that pre-pandemic 95 to 99% of people who came into my office were in one of the stages of adrenal fatigue; post pandemic I think that number is 100%.

Adrenal Fatigue

In my opinion, adrenal fatigue presents in three stages (though some say four):

Stage 1: Alarm Phase

When your body is exposed to stressors like a pandemic, job loss, or isolation, the adrenals release catecholamines (dopamine, epinephrine, and norepinephrine from the medulla) and cortisol (from the cortex).

- This is a normal response commonly known as the "fight or flight" response.

- Some typical reactions in your body are: increases in heart rate, blood pressure, and blood glucose levels; and this shuts down nonessential things like your digestion or detox processes.

- Most people will be asymptomatic.

- This should show on saliva cortisol adrenal testing as elevated cortisol and normal DHEA.

- Most of my patients have passed this phase and moved on to Stage 2.

Stage 2: Resistance Phase

When the body is repeatedly presented with stressors and it continuously releases cortisol, some doctors and scientists think a situation called "cortisol steal" can occur.

- Cortisol steal can be considered very controversial even amongst Functional Medicine doctors. Some argue for it, some against it.

- The theory comes from the fact that your adrenal hormones are all made from the same substrate, cholesterol. We all have a limited amount of cholesterol available to make hormones and it is thought that your adrenals will choose to make cortisol rather than other hormones, so under conditions of chronic stress, the cortisol will steal away the cholesterol and the production of androgens like DHEA will decrease.

- Symptoms can be things like feeling stressed, anxiety attacks, and mood swings.

- This can show up in testing as elevated and/or decreased cortisol and low DHEA.

- This is where over 90% of my patients fall.

Stage 3: Exhaustion Phase

This is adrenal insufficiency, indicating that the adrenals glands held on as long as they could but have had enough.

- Based on the reading patients have done before they come in to see me, this is where most people think they are.

- I have only seen one person clinically with true adrenal insufficiency and they had extreme toxin exposure.

- Symptoms can present as an inability to get out of bed or function, as such patients will often be bed ridden.

- True adrenal insufficiency will show up in blood testing, whereas the other stages will not, and it will show up as very low cortisol and DHEA on saliva testing.

Before we get into the testing and treatment, I would like to give my own interpretation of "adrenal fatigue." Even though I was trained as a traditional Medical Doctor who later focused on Functional Medicine, I do believe in "adrenal fatigue." So I'm an outcast in the traditional medicine world, but I am also an outcast in the Functional Medicine world because even though I will explain the testing and the supplements, I do not rely on the testing and don't believe supplements are the cure. What I believe in is that this condition stems from mental, emotional, spiritual health, trauma, anxiety, depression, family issues, relationship issues, work issues, feeling insecure, feeling not good enough, perfectionism, etc. My parents were trained doctors who grew up in Communist Poland, where it wasn't guaranteed you could eat when you were hungry; and they moved to the United States with absolutely nothing—nowhere to live, no money, no jobs and they did not speak English. They knew one person who took them into their basement, and they had to survive. Yet I grew up in Chicago with everything I could ever want: toys, friends, sports, food, fast food, candy and sugar, without a real worry, which took the problem from the physical to the mental plane. My struggle was having too much of everything and subsequently too much time in my own head. I did not struggle to survive physically the way my parents did; I struggled to survive mentally, emotionally, and spiritually. I did not do the testing but I'm pretty sure I spent most of my life in Stage 1 of adrenal fatigue, and at times it felt like Stage 2 or 3. Even though I don't think my testing would have shown that. And there is no way that taking supplements would have fixed my issues. I had to peel back the layers of my onion to figure out the root causes. Mine were being a first generation American and never feeling like I fit in or was good enough. And this is what I encourage you to do: dig deep, and uncover what is underlying. Testing and supplements can help, but if they don't, you probably have been through a lot in your life that still needs to be unpacked. In my first book, I revealed mental, emotional, spiritual health as the key to your gut health, and I believe it is the key to overall health.

I am deeply passionate about this subject despite the fact that the majority of my patients don't want to accept it or believe it. Still, they'll gladly believe in mold toxicity, heavy metals, the dangers of genetically modified foods, food sensitivities, hormone imbalances, SIBO, and dysbiosis. Which blows my mind because those things seem a lot "crazier" than believing that I'm "crazy." Your body is all connected and how you think, feel, love, and treat yourself will affect all the different organs in your body and cause them to malfunction the same way the toxins will, so why is it so hard to accept or believe? It is a daily struggle with my patients trying to convince them of this. As someone who lived in denial for many years, I get it. I also worked on the physical stuff, assuming all my health issues were due to a vitamin deficiency or toxin. But that is the easy way out—we can easily fall for the temptation to blame it on something outside of us, because dealing with the trauma we've been through is so painful. It doesn't feel good, and it frequently causes us to make dramatic life changes. One of my therapists described "change" as being as easy as peeling off your own skin… so I get it. Yet my warning to you is that you will never reach your health goals until you accept that your mental, emotional, spiritual health is the most important of all. There is a plan in *Unfunc Your Gut* on how to get started.

Now that I'm off my soapbox, let's get into testing.

Blood Tests	Reference range	Comments	Abnormalities
Cortisol	6-8 am: 10-20 mcg/dL Around 4 pm: 3-10 mcg/dL	Values decrease after you wake up.	**High cortisol** could be due to tumor, chronic stress, Cushing's disease. **Low cortisol** may be due to a problem in the pituitary gland or the adrenal gland (Addison's disease).

Blood Tests	Reference range	Comments	Abnormalities
ACTH (Adrenocorticotropic hormone) **Secreted from pituitary gland Controls release of cortisol**	10 and 60 pg/mL (at 8 AM)	• The values decrease after you wake up • < 20 pg/mL at 4 PM • 5-10 pg/mL within one hour after the usual time of falling sleep • This circadian rhythm in plasma ACTH concentrations is the cause of the parallel changes in cortisol secretion by the adrenal glands and the resulting rhythm in serum cortisol concentrations. • Your cortisol secretion is dependent on your circadian rhythm, which is why sleep is so important for your adrenal glands.[63,64]	• **Elevated** due to stress, pituitary tumor. • **Decreased** due to genetics, viruses or bacteria, tumor, injury

Blood Tests	Reference range	Comments	Abnormalities
DHEA-S (Dehydroepi-androsterone sulfate) **Most abundant hormone in body**	**Females** Ages 18 to 19: 145-395 µg/dL Ages 30 to 39: 45-270 µg/dL Ages 69 and older: 17-90 µg/dL **Males** Ages 18 to 19: 108-441 µg/dL Ages 30 to 39: 120-520 µg/dL Ages 69 and older: 28 to 175 µg/dL	• "Normal" varies by sex and decreases over time • Function not totally understood; precursor to androgens like testosterone and estrogen • Stimulates immune system[65]	• **Elevated** due to genetics, tumor, Polycystic ovarian syndrome, puberty • **Decreased** due to adrenal insufficiency (adrenal fatigue), stress, pituitary dysfunction, taking steroids
Pregnenolone	Ages >18; 33-248 ng/dL	• Precursor for androgens • First steroid hormone made • Normal for children varies by age and sex • Functions as neurotransmitter • Important role in memory and cognition • Supplementation could be used to improve memory and mood[66]	• Elevated due to tumor, Congenital Adrenal Hyperplasia (CAH) • Decreased due to adrenal insufficiency, stress • Symptoms of low pregnelenone can be poor memory, fatigue, attention deficit, dry skin, joint pain, muscle pain
Estradiol, Progesterone, Testosterone discussion (See Chapters 4 and 5)			

When first trained as a traditional M.D., I was taught to use a 24-hour urine cortisol collection when suspecting adrenal insufficiency, the theory being that because cortisol levels vary throughout the day, you collect samples over 24 hours and standardize them to a 24-hour collection, so you can identify a total cortisol deficit. This is a great test for Stage 3 of Adrenal Fatigue, but in my practice, I've only seen one person with true adrenal insufficiency. The 24-hour test will miss all cases of Stage 1 and Stage 2 adrenal fatigue and I don't think the traditional doctor cares because they don't believe in them anyway. From my perspective, Stage 3 adrenal fatigue is so rare that this test does not help me very often.

The more common testing options used in the Functional Medicine world is saliva testing, called the Adrenocortex Stress Profile—my version of a stress test! Your cardiologist will do a stress test on your heart, but Functional Medicine can assess your mental, emotional, and spiritual health, too. In an ideal world, I would not use the Adrenocortex Stress Profile frequently. I only like to order tests that change my treatment plan, and I don't need to see an imbalanced cortisol on a test to tell anyone that the focus of their health should be their mental, emotional, and spiritual health. But I use it for my patients who exhibit denial, so I do order it very frequently.

In 40 pages of intake paperwork before a patient comes in to see me, there are two questions I always focus on. Both are Yes/No questions. *Do you have an excess amount of stress in your life? Can you easily manage stress?* If someone answers No (they don't have excess stress) and Yes (they manage it easily), I know we are in for a rough time, because to me this patient is in denial. Being alive in the 2020s is excessively stressful and most people do not handle it well. In my experience, the first step is *acceptance* that we have a problem (with work, spouse, parents, or whatever it is) and that we've experienced trauma.

These things are not easy to handle. But I can't tell you how many patients sit across the desk from me and just right away say, "So, you think I'm crazy?"

Yes, I do, but I think we're all at least a little crazy—the difference is: *we are either working on it or we're not.* I explain that my job is to find the physical imbalances while your job is to do the hard work.

For the patients who resist or deny, I order the Adrenocortex Stress Profile to show them that their body is under stress and to try to motivate them to address potential, deeper issues. The test involves spitting into a tube 4 times throughout the day on a single day. We measure cortisol and DHEA levels (just in the morning). Your cortisol should start high, peak within the first hour after waking, rapidly declines over the morning hours, and then slow trend down throughout the day reaching a low at bedtime, following a bell curve on a graph.

	Reference Range	If high	If low
Cortisol 7am - 9am	0.097-0.337 mcg/dL	Could be exercise, blood sugar dysregulation, alcohol, daily stressors, medications like inhalers or creams, pain, and underlying adrenal hyperplasia or Cushing's syndrome	Decreased levels could be due to adrenal insufficiency, down regulation due to chronic stress, HPA axis dysfunction (could come from hypothalamus, pituitary gland, or adrenal glands)

	Reference Range	If high	If low
Cortisol 11am - 1pm	0.0207-0.106 mcg/dL	Conditions associated with chronic high cortisol: • Irritable Bowel Syndrome (IBS) • Leaky Gut • Dysbiosis • Chronic stress • Insomnia • Chronic migraine • Bipolar disorder • Memory Impairment • Anxiety • Depression • Premenstrual syndrome/ Premenstrual Dysphoric Disorder (PMDD) • Chronic Fatigue Syndrome (CFS)	• Conditions associated with chronic low cortisol: • Panic disorder • Suicidality • Chronic Fatigue Syndrome (CFS) • Increased CVD mortality • Depression • Lethargic • Seasonal Affective Disorder (SAD) • Postpartum depression • Panic Attacks • Generalized Anxiety Disorder • Bipolar II Disorder
Cortisol 3pm - 5pm	0.013-0.068 mcg/dL		
Cortisol 10pm - 12am	<= 0.034	Elevated levels at night are associated with insomnia, diabetes, heart disease, cancers, and osteoporosis	(See above)

	Reference Range	If high	If low
DHEA	71-640pg/mL	Elevated levels of DHEA usually reflect supplementation; other considerations include Polycystic Ovarian Syndrome (PCOS,) adrenal hyperplasia and adrenal tumors	Decreased levels can be due to advancing age, DHEA peaks at 25 years and then declines; low levels have been associated with immune dysregulation, cardiovascular disease, arthritis, osteoporosis, insomnia, declining cognition, depression, fatigue, and decreased libido
DHEA/Cortisol Ratio	358 / 2,538	An elevated ratio reflects elevated DHEA levels as compared to cortisol, which favors anabolic activity (growth)	A decreased ratio usually reflects a more catabolic (breakdown) state; it is associated with cortisol elevations and HPA-axis imbalances (HPA means hypothalamic-pituitary-adrenal)

Adrenal fatigue patterns can present in many different ways. High or low cortisol in the morning, throughout the day, or the evening. Normal DHEA with a high or low cortisol would suggest stage 1 adrenal fatigue, whereas low DHEA in the presence of high or low cortisol would suggest stage 2 adrenal fatigue; high DHEA is very rare and usually due to supplementation.

So how can you address adrenal dysfunction? The answer is different for all of us. My routine involves sleep, exercise, therapy, prayer, meditation, a gratitude list, time in nature, time with my family, and reminders on my phone to stay present and let go of control! Entire books have been written about what to do. Some of my favorites are: *The Four Agreements, Man's Search for*

Meaning, The Seven Spiritual Laws of Success, Psychocybernetics, and of course *Unfunc Your Gut.* Find the right routine for you and make your mental, emotional, and spiritual health the focus of your life. Remember some options to explore include:

Sleep

Sleep is essential for repair and recovery. The catabolic (breakdown) effects of cortisol are opposed during sleep. Chronic sleep deficit has been found in some studies[67] to significantly raise cortisol levels. Try to get 6 to 8 hours per night. Some healthy sleep habits include: avoid alcohol within 3 hours of bedtime; avoid caffeine after 2pm; assess your medication list with your doctor, as some meds can be stimulating; avoid anxiety-provoking activities like checking email or social media; plan for 8.5-9 hours in bed; and try to go to bed at the same time every day.

Some supplements that can help with sleep are melatonin (melatonin 1-5mg to go to sleep, 5-20mg of sustained release to stay asleep, 5HTP 100-200mg at night, taurine 500-2000mg at night, and magnesium glycinate 200-450mg at night.

Diet

- Shoot for 9-12 servings of vegetables and fruit per day.
- Eat the rainbow! A good practice is for every plate of food to have all the colors of the rainbow on it.
- Have frequent regular meals[68] (up to 6 per day); this helps prevent spikes in blood sugar.
- Chew food at least 30 times per mouthful; may require digestive enzymes.
- Increase fiber, minimum 35g daily.

Unfunc Your Gut

Correlational studies[69] have shown that the microbiome in people with anxiety or depression differs from healthy controls. Promoting the growth of commensal bacteria, particularly probiotic strains such as Lactobacilli, may correlate with increased emotional resilience under stress.

Exercise

Exercise increases endorphin levels and improves mood, improves circulation, reduces anxiety,[70] reduces depression, and improves quality of sleep by lowering cortisol and heart rate in response to stress. Alternative type exercises like yoga[71] and tai chi can elicit the relaxation response.

Breathwork

4-7-8 Breathing. Do 4 cycles 2 times per day. First, let your lips part. Make a whooshing sound, exhaling completely through your mouth. Next, close your lips, inhaling silently through your nose as you count to four in your head. Then, for seven seconds, hold your breath. Make another whooshing exhale from your mouth for eight seconds.

Belly breathing. This slows the heartbeat and can lower or stabilize blood pressure. Lie on your back on a flat surface with your knees bent. You can use a pillow under your head and your knees for support, if that's more comfortable. Place one hand on your upper chest and the other on your belly, just below your rib cage. Breathe in slowly through your nose, letting the air in deeply, towards your lower belly. The hand on your chest should remain still, while the one on your belly should rise. Tighten your abdominal muscles and let them fall inward as you exhale through pursed lips. The hand on your belly should move down to its original position. Practice for 5 to 10 minutes, 3 to 4 times a day, if possible.

Daily Habits

Laugh. One of my favorite motivational speeches that brings me to tears every year is Coach Jim Valvano's acceptance speech for the Arthur Ashe Courage and Humanitarian Award (Jimmy V was fighting cancer and passed away not long after this speech). Here is an excerpt:

> "When people say to me, how do you get through life, or each day? It's the same thing. To me, there are three things we all should do every day. We should do this every day of our lives. Number 1 is laugh. You should laugh every day. Number 2 is think. You should spend some time in thought. Number 3 is you should have your emotions moved to tears, could be happiness or joy. But think about it. If you laugh, you think and you cry, that's a full day. That's a heckuva day. You do that seven days a week, you're going to have something special. I know, I gotta go, I gotta go. And I got one last thing, and I said it before, and I'm gonna say it again: Cancer can take away all my physical abilities. It cannot touch my mind, it cannot touch my heart, and it cannot touch my soul. And those three things are going to carry on forever."

Sing. A single hour of singing was associated with increases in mood and a decrease in cortisol.[72]

Prayer/meditation/mindfulness. In a 10-year study, religious participation predicted steeper, "healthier" cortisol slopes at the 10-year follow-up.[73] Find the right balance for you. I believe in God and pray, but if you do not that is OK, and maybe you will do better to focus on meditation and mindfulness. I like to incorporate all of them.

Let go of control. Don't try to force things. If you set yourself a goal, do everything in your power to achieve that goal, but once all your work has been done, let it go and trust that however it is supposed to work out, it will work out.

Heart Rate Variability (HRV)

HRV is a measure of the beat-to-beat fluctuations in heart rate. The heart can go faster or slower depending on which nervous system response is activated. The rhythm of a healthy heart is surprisingly irregular, with the time interval between consecutive heart beats constantly changing. This is totally normal and the variability is due to the balance between your Sympathetic Nervous System (fight or flight, faster heart) and Parasympathetic Nervous System (rest and digest, slower heart). So when we are stressed, the heart goes faster and when we are relaxed the heart goes slower. HRV is a way to slow down! Which most of us, including myself, need. HRV programs typically use imagery and one study compared control imagery versus compassion imagery, with the participants in the compassion imagery group showing a lower salivary cortisol result along with an increase in HRV.[74]

Neurofeedback

A similar practice to HRV except for the brain instead of the heart is neurofeedback. Neurofeedback is also called EEG Biofeedback, because it is based on electrical brain activity, the electroencephalogram, or (EEG), which measures your brain waves. Practicing neurofeedback can teach the brain to function more efficiently. Just like HRV the person can see how their brain is working and learn how to address imbalanced patterns. This is a gradual learning process, again just like all aspects of our mental, emotional, and spiritual health.

EMDR

EMDR (Eye Movement Desensitization and Reprocessing) is a psychotherapy that enables people to heal from trauma. It is my therapy of choice for trauma, and my definition of trauma is *anything less than nurturing.* EMDR is believed to work through biological mechanisms involved in Rapid Eye Movement (REM) sleep; internal associations arise, and the person begins to process the traumatic memory. When successful the meaning of painful events is transformed on an emotional level. I highly, highly recommend it. Brainspotting is a similar technique but instead of bilateral stimulation like EMDR, brain spotting focuses the eye on a fixed-gaze position.

Psychotherapy

I listed a few different types of therapy above, but there are many types of therapy: cognitive behavioral therapy (CBT), dialectical behavior therapy (DBT), and psychodynamic therapy, just to name a few. If you aren't sure where to begin, call a local therapy practice to discuss the options.

Fellowship

Some fellowship groups include church and Twelve-Step groups. A meta-analytic review of 148 studies on over 300,000 people found that people who were more socially connected were 50 percent less likely to die over a given period.[75] I am not advising you to disregard the advice of health organizations—everyone must keep themselves and others safe; I am just making a point that excessive isolation is not good for mental health. The good news is that these groups are now conducted regularly via Zoom. If you have never been to a group like this, don't be scared; you are walking into a room of people who have probably been through worse and are fighting to get better. Keep exploring until you find the right group or groups for you.

Supplements

This is yet another area where I could disagree with traditional, and even some alternative doctors. There are a number of alternative practitioners out there diagnosing their patients with adrenal fatigue, and then prescribing them large, expensive supplement protocols and selling them on the hope that the supplements will be the magic cure. This is a traditional medicine approach, a pill for the ill. In my experience, adrenal fatigue will never heal if you don't dig deep into the underlying traumas and pain, no matter how many supplements you take. Here's a look at supplements that can be helpful in healing, but remember: they are not the cure.

Supplements	Function	Dosing
B-complex[76,77,78]	Are co-factors in hormone production	B5 (pantothenic acid) 1000-1500 mg B6 (pyridoxine) 50-100 mg Biotin 1000 mcg) Folate 400-800 mcg
Vitamin C	Needed to produce cortisol	1 gram 3x daily
Magnesium (usually glycinate for calming effects)	• Catalyst for >200 chemical reactions in body • Magnesium deficiency intensifies adverse reactions to stress	400-600mg daily
Omega-3 EPA/DHA[79,80,81]	• Can decrease excess adrenal activation • Epinephrine, cortisol, and energy expenditure can all be decreased with supplementation • Omega-3 deficiency adversely affects learning and cognitive behavior	1-3 grams daily
Zinc	• >300 human enzymes utilize zinc • Under conditions of major stress, zinc is lost in urine, sweat, saliva, and plasma concentrations • Zinc has anti-depressant effects; low zinc levels can function as a biomarker for depression • Zinc deficiency leads to decreased zinc in the nerve synapses, resulting in a decrease of GABA and a rise in glutamate causing excitotoxicity and may be contribute to anxiety, depression, and bipolar disorder [82,83,84,85]	20-50mg daily

Supplements	Function	Dosing
DHEA	• Many people take DHEA under the thought process it would be converted to testosterone, but it is has not been shown to be an effective testosterone treatment. • DHEA is thought to have its own receptors that give it some benefit, specifically DHEA has been found to have positive effects on cardiovascular health[86]	Females: 5-25mg twice daily Males: 10-50mg twice daily

Adrenal Extract

There are a number of supplement companies which make an adrenal extract (it should be typically advertised as the extract of bovine adrenal gland). These could be helpful but you should be aware that you are taking hormones. In a study, the researchers purchased the 12 most popular dietary supplements that patients take for adrenal support.[87] They found that all 12 supplements contained a detectable amount of triiodothyronine (T3- thyroid hormone), with daily exposure of up to 1322 ng. Additionally, a substantial number of supplements also contained a variety of adrenal hormones ranging from a daily exposure of 1231.2 ng for pregnenolone (most common) to 159.32 ng for cortisone (least common). (None of the OTC supplements declared on their label that they contained thyroid or adrenal hormones.) Not great, and this is why supplements can get a bad rep from traditional medicine. These supplements may be helpful, but you should just be aware what you're taking.

Adaptogens

Adaptogens are herbs or fungi that help our bodies to react to or to recover from stress, and could boost immunity and overall well-being. Some studies have shown that adaptogens can combat fatigue, enhance mental performance, ease depression and anxiety, and help you thrive.[88] It is thought that they work through an effect in maintaining HPA-axis homeostasis. Ashwagandhah can be traced back as many as 6,000 years in Ayurvedic Medicine, and we will also look at a few others.

Adaptogens	Function	Dose
Ashwagandha	• Also known as Indian Ginseng and comes from an evergreen shrub that's found in India, Africa and parts of the Middle East • Traditionally used for: stress tolerance, vigor and stamina, convalescence, nervous exhaustion, fatigue, geriatric debility, physical and mental stress, and insomnia. • Supports cognitive function, reasoning, and critical thinking [89,90,91]	500 - 3000mg per day
Theanine	• Comes from green, black and white tea • Calms sympathetic response to stress • Associated with decreased heart rate, decreased cortisol, increases dopamine and serotonin levels [92,93,94]	600 - 1200mg at night
St John's Wort	• Demonstrated similar efficacy to SSRIs in factors that decrease in symptoms, remission rate, and relapse rates in patients with mild to moderate depression[95]	600mg per day

Adaptogens	Function	Dose
Rhodiola	• Positively impacted overall mood through regulating cell response to stress • Decreased depression and anxiety symptoms including insomnia, somatization and emotional instability	340mg per day
Panax Ginseng	• Traditionally used to stimulate mental and physical activity, enhance stamina, prevent fatigue, and increase resistance to stress • Considered the most valued and widely used herb in China and Asia • Anti-anxiety effects • Improves cortisol/DHEA ratios and stimulates the immune system, increasing activity of natural killer cells	100 - 200mg twice daily

Never start any supplements without first consulting your doctor. Remember, if you do try supplements or adaptogens you will usually need to take them for 6 to 12 weeks to see results.

CHAPTER 3

The Pancreas

The pancreas is located in the abdomen behind the stomach and has two main functions, labeled as exocrine and endocrine function. The organ is spongy, about six to ten inches long, and shaped like a flat pear. Anatomically, the pancreas is said to have a head, neck, body, and tail.

The exocrine function of the pancreas is to aid in digestion. Almost all of the pancreas (about 95%) consists of exocrine tissue that produces pancreatic enzymes for digestion. (We covered the exocrine function of the pancreas in *Unfunc Your Gut*.) Since this a book about hormones, we are going to focus on the endocrine function, which is made up of cells called islets of Langerhans. Even though only 5% of the pancreas is responsible for endocrine function, I would argue that this 5% is even more important than the other 95%, because *the endocrine function is responsible for regulating blood sugar.* There are two main enzymes that control blood sugar: insulin that lowers blood sugar and glucagon which raises blood sugar. In the United States, we have become all too familiar with insulin, but we don't hear much about glucagon. We will get into why and what you can do to understand the dynamics of insulin, glucagon, and blood sugar balance. Since this is also a book about toxins, before we dive into the endocrine function, I would like to talk about pancreatitis.

Pancreatitis

Pancreatitis is simply inflammation of the pancreas. The pancreas becomes inflamed when the enzymes it secretes start destroying the organ itself. It can happen acutely, lasting just a matter of days, or it can become chronic. It is twice as common in adult men and is rare in children; about 87,000 people per year are diagnosed with pancreatitis, so it is pretty rare. Symptoms of pancreatitis are typically severe, steady pain in the upper middle part of the abdomen, but the key distinguishing factor from a stomachache is that the pain associated with pancreatitis typically radiates to the back. It can also present with jaundice (yellowing of the skin) and a low-grade fever.

The most common causes of pancreatitis are gallstones and alcohol abuse, but other causes include medications (more than 85 drugs have been associated with pancreatitis, like traditional birth control/oral contraceptives or diuretics used for high blood pressure), elevated triglycerides, infections (viruses and parasites), and it also can be autoimmune.[96] Treatment usually involves hospitalization and making the patient NPO (nothing per mouth) for a few days. The person is given nutrition support intravenously (IV) and usually strong pain medications like opiates; and sometimes they are given antibiotics as well.

So, why is pancreatitis such a relevant discussion in a book about hormones and toxins? Functional medicine is all about the underlying cause, therefore we are thinking about why someone would get gallstones, high triglycerides, or autoimmune disease, for example. In all of these cases, the first place I would look is toxins. An important reminder here is that toxins are not just heavy metals, mold, or glyphosate. Your food can be a harmful toxin, as can a bad relationship and an imbalanced microbiome. When these toxins are present and your bucket starts to fill up or overflow, they can present as disease just about anywhere in the body.

Let's say you follow the standard American diet (SAD) for 40 years and think this is totally normal. The SAD comes from school and what is marketed on TV and in the media. We learn that eating pancakes with orange juice is a good breakfast, macaroni and cheese is delicious for lunch, and pizza makes a great dinner, as long as it comes with a dessert of ice cream or cheesecake. The SAD diet consists of high intakes of animals, which themselves are not being fed well, processed meat (e.g., hot dogs and deli meats), canned and pre-packaged foods, butter, sugar, fried foods available at almost any drive-thru, high-fat dairy products, eggs, refined grains, potatoes, corn (which includes high-fructose corn syrup) and high-sugar drinks like sodas or pop, depending where you are from.[97] This is a toxic diet, and yet it's considered the norm. In fact, it is what I inspired to, being an immigrant and wanting to fit in with my classmates.

Due to the upside-down food pyramid, as well as the Seven Countries Study that recommended people to eat 6 to 11 servings of bread, cereal, rice, and pasta per day and to only use fats sparingly, fat was removed from food and replaced with sugar. This phenomenon will lead us into the discussion of the endocrine function of the pancreas soon. The problem is that once sugar is in our body, it is either used or if there is too much, it is stored. *What is it stored as,* you ask? As fat, known as triglycerides.

The shocking part is that even though fat was vilified and replaced with sugar, somehow the American diet still consists of 35% fat.[98] We are talking about pancreatitis, and one of its greatest causes is gallstones. Over 3 million cases of gallstones are diagnosed each year in the United States. Gallstones are hardened deposits (stones) of digestive fluid, usually made up of mostly cholesterol. Gallstones can vary in size and number and may or may not cause symptoms. Bile from the gallbladder and pancreatic enzymes pass through the same tube called the bile duct. And if gallstones have built up in the gallbladder, they can be released from the gallbladder and can block the duct. When this happens, the enzymes released from the pancreas build up and eat the pancreas itself instead of digesting your food. I know, nasty stuff!

So what causes gallstones? Studies suggest it is a diet high in fat, a.k.a. the SAD diet. In 2010, researchers looked at 305 women in Iran (note: gallstones are more common in women, aged 40 plus, with obesity, who have had children or taken hormones like contraceptives), and compared diet to risk of gallstones. They defined *healthy diet* as high amounts of vegetables, fruits, low-fat dairy products, nuts, whole grains, legumes, fish and spices, and low intake of salt, compared with an *unhealthy diet* that has a high intake of refined grain, sugar, red meat, soft drinks, snacks, processed meats, high-fat dairy products, and eggs. They found gallstone risk to be increased in the group of women following the "unhealthy diet."[99] Other studies have found the vegetarian diet to be protective against gallstones.[100] Since you need a surgeon to remove a gallstone in case it is blocked, I would recommend a Functional medicine doctor to help you prevent gallstones from forming or coming back instead. An easy way to start is to eat 9 to 12 servings of vegetables and fruit per day.

Insulin

There are two hormones you don't want too much of. The first one is cortisol, which we learned about in Chapter 2, the other is insulin. My mentor, colleague, and friend Dr. Dan Luckazer wrote that *insulin insensitivity* (which causes high blood sugar) may be the single most important underlying metabolic dysfunction related to chronic disease; the kidneys, eyes, nerves, and blood vessels are typically most affected. Now, let's learn the basics of insulin and sugar, and then we can discuss what can go wrong and how to fix it.[101]

The role of insulin is to maintain the blood sugar (glucose) level in your blood. It's like a key to let glucose enter your cells all over the body. When you eat, your body breaks food down in the gut tube so that we can absorb the nutrients and sugar into our body; yet only once they cross the gut barrier (and are now in the blood) are they actually "in your body." Insulin then helps move the sugar from the blood into your cells. When sugar enters your cells, it is either used as fuel for energy right away or stored for later use (as fat). The functions of insulin are to regulate cellular energy supply and macronutrient balance, and also to direct anabolic processes—which means, it makes things grow. Insulin also stops the breakdown of fat. When there is no sugar coming in from the diet, glucagon (the other main hormone in sugar balance) causes you to break down stored fat for energy.

Your body is very smart. When you give it energy through your diet, it uses it efficiently and stores the rest in case food becomes scarce, in which case it will use what's stored to survive. This system of using food as energy and storing the rest was a key to our survival, but through human abundance and food manufacturing, diets high in sugar, fat, soda, and processed foods have put this system under extreme strain. In 1980, 4.8 percent of men and 7.9 percent of U.S. women were obese;[102] by 2000, the obesity rate was 30.5%; and by 2018 it was 42.4%.[103] That's a sharp increase in a short amount of time.

What changed during those years? Our diet—the most important factor in determining the amount of sugar in your blood. As we learned in *Unfunc Your Gut*, "Based on current research, the average American consumes 276,000 calories (152 pounds) per year in added sugar, whereas in 1980 it was 72,640 calories (40 pounds)."[104] That's nearly four times the sugar!

As the sugar increased so did our weight, along with the diseases associated with it.

Your pancreas is prepared to release a set amount of insulin, but it was not prepared for 152 pounds of sugar per year. The good news is: it can make more when it needs too. The bad news is: you can't make more insulin receptors, which leads to insulin resistance.

Insulin Resistance

Insulin resistance eoccurs when a normal or elevated insulin level produces a low response… in other words, when insulin doesn't do its job as effectively. When the pancreas detects this, so it completely makes more. I originally studied Economics in college and this concept reminds me of the Law of Diminishing Returns, which states that in productive processes, increasing a factor of production by one unit, while holding all other production factors constant, will at some point return a lower unit of output per incremental unit of input. In other words, if increasing a variable increases the outcome, this doesn't mean it will continue to; at some point a direct correlation between the two factors may eventually become inversely correlated. Due to chronic high sugar intake, more insulin is released, and in turn it becomes less effective. This is insulin resistance.

Many people can remain in this state for years and not develop Diabetes Mellitus II. Type I Diabetes is when someone's pancreas cannot make enough insulin, a condition that usually starts in childhood, but we will focus on Type II, which starts in adults who eat too much sugar, leading to insulin resistance, where eventually the pancreas cannot keep up and insulin receptors cease to function properly.

Pre-diabetes

When your blood sugar is elevated but not high enough to diagnose diabetes, pre-diabetes ensues. According to the CDC, more than 84% of people with pre-diabetes do not know they have it.[105] This is because there are no symptoms that someone with pre-diabetes would feel. The most shocking number to me is that 1 in 3 adults in the United States have pre-diabetes, about 88 million people.[106] In my opinion, this is because people do not understand how toxic the Standard American Diet (SAD) is. Society relies on the ease of obtaining fast and processed food, and is basically numb to the constant onslaught of marketing promoting these unhealthy foods. The risk factors for pre-diabetes are: excess weight, physical inactivity, smoking, large amounts of alcohol, sleep issues, high cholesterol, and high blood pressure. Let's look at how pre-diabetes affects different tissues in the body.

Affected Tissue	Consequences
Muscle	Muscle accounts for 60 to 70% of insulin uptake. Under normal conditions, insulin promotes glycogen synthesis, which allows energy to be released. In insulin resistance, glycogen synthesis is impaired, leading to impaired energy production. Think fatigue, exercise intolerance, weakness.[107]
Adipose (a.k.a. fat)	Adipose accounts for about 10% of insulin uptake. Insulin promotes lipogenesis (the growth of fat) and suppresses lipolysis (stops the breakdown of fat).[108]
Liver	Insulin is key to many metabolic processes in the liver. In insulin resistance, the liver makes more fat leading to high triglycerides.

Affected Tissue	Consequences
Blood Vessels	Insulin plays many roles on our blood vessels (other ways they can be described are as endothelium or vasculature). Insulin resistance causes the arteries to be more constricted which leads to high blood pressure. The blood becomes more likely to clot (think heart attack and stroke).
Brain	Insulin receptors have been found in many regions of the brain. Insulin is believed to act as a neuropeptide, involved in satiety (feeling full), appetite regulation, olfaction (smell), memory and cognition. In the Functional Medicine world, we call dementia "type III diabetes," given insulin's role in normal cognitive functioning and in the regulation of plaques that are found in dementia patients.[109,110]
Kidney	Insulin regulates mineral transport and gluconeogenisis in the kidneys. Insulin can decrease sodium excretion, contributing to high blood pressure. Chronic high sugar severely damages the kidneys, which is why you see so many diabetics on dialysis (a treatment where machines do the job of the kidneys).[111]
Ovaries	Insulin causes the ovaries to make more hormones, including estrogen. One study suggested that the frequency of PCOS was 18.33%.[112] Symptoms of PCOS (Polycystic Ovary Syndrome) can include irregular periods, excess facial hair, thinning hair, cysts on the ovaries, and infertility. Some have suggested that all women with PCOS should be treated for insulin resistance.[113]

Those are the different tissues that are affected, but you may be more familiar with the diseases that result when those tissues are affected. Pre-COVID in 2019, the most common causes of death[114] were as follows:

- Heart disease
- Cancer
- Accidents
- Stroke
- Chronic lower respiratory diseases
- Alzheimer disease
- Diabetes mellitus

- Kidney disease
- Influenza and pneumonia
- Suicide
- Chronic liver disease

- Septicemia (widespread infection)
- Hypertension
- Parkinson disease

What do the overwhelming majority of those conditions have in common? Diet and lifestyle. Sugar = insulin = fat growth = obesity = heart disease, stroke, Alzheimer's disease, Diabetes mellitus, kidney disease, chronic liver disease, septicemia, hypertension. The connection with sugar and those diseases probably makes sense. Here's one that you may not believe, but research has shown that being overweight or obese increases the risk of 11 types of cancers including colorectal, postmenopausal breast, ovarian, and pancreatic cancer.

Fast forward to 2 years post Covid and number three on the list is now COVID-19. One study found that 40% of COVID-19 deaths were in people with diabetes.[115] What's more, 1 out of 10 people with diabetes die within one week, making the mortality rate three times higher than that of the overall population.[116] The craziest part of these statistics is that these numbers do not include pre-diabetics, who make up one third of the population. The numbers aren't available because, as we learned, most people with pre-diabetes don't know they have it; it is not assessed and reported in that data. Might the number jump as high as 70% of COVID-19 deaths are related to blood sugar and insulin? Could it be higher?

What if we shut down sugar instead of everything else? It saddens and frustrates me that the mainstream media focuses on scaring people instead of offering tools to heal. The good news is, even if you have insulin resistance, pre-diabetes, or diabetes type II, there is hope for you. These conditions are reversible, you just have to put in the work. There will always be the pharmaceutical industry for those who are not ready to change, but for those who don't want to rely on them, there is a path forward. Get the func out!

Diabetes

When your blood sugar gets too high and stays high, that is diabetes. About 90 to 95% of people with diabetes have type II. With type II diabetes, your insulin is less effective and the body can't keep blood sugar at normal levels. Diabetes typically develops over many years, but more and more is being seen in children and teens. Approximately 5 to 10% of the people who have diabetes have type I. Type I diabetes is thought to be caused by an autoimmune reaction that stops your body from making insulin. It is usually diagnosed in children, teens, and young adults. People with type I need to take insulin every day to survive.

The major problem with diabetes is that it affects the entire body, as I mentioned above. In my opinion, elevated blood sugar and all the consequences due to it is the biggest pandemic we are dealing with. Did you know that healthcare costs are 2.3 times higher for diabetics? And that the annual cost of diagnosed diabetics in America is $327 billion,[117] and that one out of every four dollars in U.S. health care is spent on people with diabetes? The difference is that we are not doing anything about this pandemic. The same processed, artificial, sugar-filled food is given to children in schools; our grocery aisles are full of food with sugar; and the marketing of these foods on TV and media is staggering—and ignored. Who is benefitting from this?

Here is the bigger problem with those numbers: 90 to 95% of these people have type II diabetes, which mostly onsets because of "lifestyle choices." Lifestyle choices are preventable factors that are fully in someone's control. There is a genetic factor in some bodies, but our genes are not our destiny. Even if you have a genetic mutation that predisposes you or increases your risk of developing diabetes, this does not mean that you have to develop diabetes. The determining factor will be your lifestyle.

Let's look at some lab testing and then we will jump into what changes you can make.

Lab Testing for Diabetes

	Normal Range	Pre-Diabetes	Diabetes
Fasting Blood Sugar	70 - 99 mg/dl	100 - 125 mg/dL	>126 mg/dl
Hemoglobin A1C	4 - 5.6%	5.7 - 6.4%	>6.5%
Oral Glucose Tolerance test	<140 mg/dl	140 - 199 mg/dL	>200mg/dl[118]

When testing for diabetes, a *fasting blood sugar test* is drawn after 8 hours of not eating in addition to a previous 8-hour overnight fast. Hemoglobin A1C measures the percentage of blood sugar attached to hemoglobin and it indicates your average blood sugar level for the past two to three months. For example, an A1C level between 5.7 and 6.4% indicates an average blood sugar of 117 to 137 mg/dl whereas a A1C of 7% indicates and average blood glucose of 153mg/dl.

An *oral glucose tolerance* test is when they test your body's response to sugar. You'll drink a syrupy liquid containing 75 grams of sugar. Your serum glucose level is checked 2 hours later. If the numbers are high or out of range, this indicates your insulin is not working.

Fasting Insulin

There is a number that I prefer to screen my patients for, one that is not used in traditional medicine. Using a *fasting insulin test*, we measure the insulin levels after an overnight fast of 8 hours. I order the other traditional labs as well, but I call fasting insulin levels my "pre- pre- diabetes test." We just learned what insulin resistance or diabetes type II is: your body releases more and more insulin to counteract the high sugar levels, and the insulin becomes less effective, so more is released. So would it not make sense that insulin levels are usually elevated before there are abnormalities in blood sugar levels?[119] That's why a blood sugar test might come back completely normal even if you are suffering from insulin resistance. Your insulin levels, however, will be elevated.

All this considered, this test is not perfect. There can be variations in fasting insulin, but for someone who wants to get ahead of the game, I would recommend having your doctor measure your fasting insulin levels as part of your screening.

Fasting insulin normal range is about 2 to 19.6 mIU/mL. Researcher Stephen Guyenet wrote that the average insulin level in the United States is 8.8 mIU/ml for men and 8.4 for women. Another study on 965 people found that if fasting insulin levels were used as a screening test, a value greater than 9.0 mIU/mL, would correctly identify pre-diabetes in 80% of affected patients.[120] This is why I give my patients a goal of between 2 to 6 to minimize their risk of insulin resistance and type II diabetes.

Why your traditional doctor doesn't use this number as part of your evaluation I do not know. The traditional medical model is based on getting people sick at a young age and then keeping them alive and sick as long as possible; it is endless profits with a customer for life. In contrast, the Functional Medicine model is: find out as much information as possible in the beginning, implement significant interventions, spend more money upfront, and then stay out of the doctor's office. It is a terrible "business" model for doctors. I usually have a few visits with a patient in the first 6 to 12 months, and then I only hear from them when they want to say "hi" or if they refer a friend or family member, for which I am always grateful. We are really "getting the func out."

So, what can you do to get your blood sugar under control?

The easiest and fastest ways are diet and exercise, both of which we dove deeply into with *Unfunc Your Gut,* so I would recommend reviewing that. In the meantime, I will give you my fundamental recommendations here: eat 9 to 12 servings of vegetables and fruit per day and cut out added sugar. There won't be room for the other junk if you do! Or start following a Mediterranean diet, which has been found to decrease diabetes risk by 83%.[121] There are many renditions of the Mediterranean diet, but in general it refers a diet high in vegetables, fruits, legumes, nuts, beans, cereals, whole grains, fish, and unsaturated fats such as olive oil. It usually includes a low intake of meat and dairy. It is low in refined grains, such as white bread, white pasta, and pizza dough containing white flour; refined oils (including canola oil and soybean oil); foods with added sugars, such as pastries, sodas, and candies; and deli meats, hot dogs, and other processed meats. Another dietary tool I previously discussed at length in *Unfunc Your Gut* was intermittent fasting. I suggest that everyone include intermittent fasting in their routine. I recommend 24 to 36 hours, 2 to 3 times per week.

Any of the tips discussed in the adrenal chapter will also be effective in lowering blood sugar levels. There are a few supplements that can be very helpful as well, including:

	Daily Dose	
Alpha Lipoic Acid	600 - 1200mg	• Improves insulin sensitivity • Enhances glucose uptake • Is an antioxidant • Increases other antioxidants[122]

	Daily Dose	
Chromium	1,000 mcg	• Improves Insulin function
Berberine	1,000 - 1,500 mg	• Increases insulin sensitivity • Promotes insulin production • Regulates metabolism • Increases breakdown of glucose • Increases nitric oxide (NO) production, which helps widen arteries • Slows carbohydrate absorption from the gut[123]
CoQ10	100 - 200mg	• Improves blood sugar control • Improves vascular function[124]
Vitamin C	500 - 1,000mg	• Lowers blood sugar and blood pressure • Is an antioxidant[125]
Zinc	15-20mg	• Decreases fasting glucose[126]
Selenium	200mcg	• Improves blood sugar • Is an antioxidant[127]
EPA/DHA (fish oil)	1,000mg	• Improves insulin resistance[128]
Magnesium	200 - 400mg	• Lowers blood sugar • Improves insulin sensitivity[129]
Vitamin D	Dose based on your levels, usually between 2,000 - 10,000iu daily	• Increases insulin sensitivity[130]

Important: Never rely on just supplements and never start any without first talking to your healthcare practitioner. The bad news is that diabetes or insulin resistance is, in my opinion, the greatest health crisis our world faces. The good news is that it is totally in your control.

CHAPTER 4

Female Hormones

I never imagined I would be writing a chapter about female reproductive (sex) hormones. Ever since I was young, girls made me nervous and I always felt insecure. Then, when I was going through medical school and learning about female hormones, I thought to myself, no wonder women are so complex. Now having helped women with hormonal imbalances for more than 10 years, I find it comforting to write this in the hopes of helping you.

The main female hormones that we will discuss are estrogen and progesterone. Women also make some testosterone, though less than men, and we will dive deeper into testosterone in the following chapter. Hormones are important to understand because they affect many different parts of our body.

In both males and females, sex hormones are involved in:

- puberty and sexual development
- reproduction
- sexual desire
- regulating bone and muscle growth
- inflammatory responses
- regulating cholesterol levels
- promoting hair growth
- body fat distribution

Reproductive hormone levels fluctuate throughout a person's life. Factors that can affect the levels of female sex hormones include:

- age
- menstruation
- pregnancy
- menopause

- stress
- medications
- environment

Estrogen

The majority of estrogen production occurs in the ovaries, and some is produced by the adrenal glands. But the most interesting place estrogen production occurs is in adipose (fat cells). (Remember how we learned that science suggests all women diagnosed with PCOS should be treated as type II diabetics? PCOS is commonly associated with excess adipose tissue, which can make more estrogen, onsetting or worsening PCOS and then making it more difficult to lose weight.[131]

Estrogen plays a crucial role in reproductive and sexual development, which begins when a woman reaches puberty. Estrogen also plays a role in protecting the heart from cholesterol, regulates cholesterol production in the liver, increases bone strength and density, has an anti-aging effect on skin, helps the brain with body temperature regulation, memory function, and influences sex drive. When puberty starts (age 8 to 13) it promotes the growth of the breasts, pubic and underarm hair, and signals the start of menstrual cycles. Then estrogen continues to play a role within the ovaries, stimulating maturation and ovulation, and also prepares the uterus monthly for pregnancy or the menstrual cycle.

There are estrogen receptors in the central nervous system (CNS), blood vessels, lungs, heart, kidneys, uterus, breasts, liver, gut, ovaries, bladder, and bones. Imbalances in estrogen could have an effect on any of these parts of the body.

There are three types of estrogen: Estrone (E1) is the main type of estrogen present in the body after menopause, made primarily in fat cells. Estradiol (E2) is the strongest estrogen, made by the ovaries and present in the body before menopause; this the one a woman is most familiar with. Estriol (E3) is the least potent estrogen, present in the body primarily during pregnancy.

The way estrogen is broken down is also very important. It is metabolized in two major pathways, broken down into 2-hydroxyestrone (2-OH) and into 16-hydroxyestrone (16-OH), with a small amount metabolized into 4-hydroxyestrone (4-OH). Each of these metabolites has distinct functions in the body. The metabolite 2-hydroxyestrone (2-OH) has multiple health benefits, working to block stronger estrogens that promote cell proliferation and possible cancer growth. Conversely,16-OH increases cell proliferation. Higher levels of 16-OH are associated with inflammation;[132] the breakdown favoring 16-OH instead of 2-OH can be due to things like excess levels of omega-6 fatty acids (bad fats from your diet), obesity, hypothyroidism, and toxins. These types of toxins would also favor breakdown into 4-OH, which is thought to promote cancer by damaging DNA. You can measure how your estrogen is being broken down via urine testing.

Progesterone

Progesterone is made in the ovaries, adrenal glands, and placenta. Progesterone is produced during ovulation (it starts around day 14 of your cycle, when you count day 1 as the first day of bleeding) and a lot is produced during pregnancy.

Progesterone helps stabilize the menstrual cycle, but its main job is to get the uterus ready for pregnancy by helping thicken the lining of the uterus to prepare for a fertilized egg. It also stops muscle contractions in the uterus that would cause the body to reject an egg. If there is no fertilized egg, then when progesterone levels drop, menstruation begins. If pregnancy occurs, progesterone continues to be produced and stimulates blood vessels in the uterus that will allow nutrients to get to the fetus. Once the placenta develops at about 8 to 12 weeks of pregnancy, it also begins to secrete progesterone. Progesterone remains elevated throughout pregnancy, so the body does not produce more eggs. It also helps prepare the breasts for milk production. Having a low progesterone can lead to irregular periods, difficulty conceiving, and a higher risk of complications during pregnancy. There are no known serious medical consequences due to the body making too much progesterone.

LH and FSH

Luteinizing hormone (LH) and follicle-stimulating hormone (FSH) are called gonadotropins because they stimulate the gonads (the testes in males, and the ovaries in females) to make hormones. These hormones come from the same place that TSH for your thyroid comes from and ACTH for your adrenal glands—that is, your pituitary gland in your brain. The function of these hormones is to stimulate the ovaries to produce estrogen and progesterone. The ovaries will produce estradiol during the follicular phase and progesterone during luteal phase

Both surge in the middle of the cycle and trigger ovulation. These levels are more commonly in balance than the estrogen and progesterone is.

The Menstrual Cycle

The menstrual cycle is divided into 3 phases: the follicular (before release of the egg), the ovulatory (egg release), and the luteal (after egg release) phases. The average duration of a menstrual cycle is 28 days, with most cycle lengths between 25 to 30 days.[133]

A cycle which is less than 21 days is termed polymenorrheic, while menstrual cycles greater than 35 days, are termed oligomenorrheic. Women have approximately 35 years of regular, predictable menstrual cycles. The menstrual cycle is typically most abnormal at the beginning of reproductive life (menarche) and at the end (menopause).

Follicular Phase

The first day of a period (first day of bleeding) starts a new menstrual cycle. Estrogen and progesterone levels are very low at this point, and this can cause irritability and mood changes. The pituitary gland releases FSH and LH, which increase estrogen levels, and signals follicle growth in the ovaries. A follicle is a small sac of fluid in the ovaries that contains one developing egg. At about day 8, one dominant follicle will emerge in each ovary and the ovaries will absorb the remaining follicles. As the follicle continues growing, it will produce more estrogen, which stimulates the release of endorphins that raise energy levels and improve mood (i.e., a woman may feel down and depressed, and then a couple days later happy and energetic, just due to normal hormonal changes). Estrogen supports the endometrium, which is the lining of the uterus, in case pregnancy occurs. The length of the follicular phase can range from 10 to 16 days, a variance which creates the different time lengths for the cycle.

Ovulatory Phase

This shortest phase, which only lasts about 24 hours, happens when the egg is released.

During the ovulatory phase, estrogen and LH levels in the body peak, causing a follicle to burst and release its egg from the ovary. The egg travels from the ovary through the fallopian tube and into the uterus. An egg can survive for around 12 to 24 hours after leaving the ovary. Fertilization of the egg can only occur during this phase and usually happens while the egg is moving through the fallopian tubes.

Luteal Phase

The ruptured follicle releases progesterone, which thickens the uterine lining, preparing it to receive a fertilized egg. Once the egg reaches the end of the fallopian tube, it attaches to the uterine wall. If the egg that attaches is fertilized, progesterone will be released. If an unfertilized egg attaches, it will cause estrogen and progesterone levels to decline. This marks the beginning of the premenstrual week. The luteal phase of the cycle is relatively constant in all women, with a duration of 14 days.

And there you have it, a woman's hormones and cycle simplified in a few pages. Easy, right? So how does it get complicated? When should a woman consider the possibility of an imbalance in her hormones?

Symptoms of a hormonal imbalance could be:

- Mood swings
- Breast tenderness
- Heavy periods/cramps
- Anxiety
- Fatigue
- Sleep disruption
- Hot flashes
- Low libido
- PCOS
- Acne

- Infertility
- Hirsutism
- Weight gain
- Hair loss
- Brain fog

- Endometriosis
- Uterine fibroids
- Irritable bowel symptoms (diarrhea, constipation, both, abdominal pain, bloating, etc.)

Many listed here symptoms overlap with symptoms we saw in the previous chapters, which again shows the importance of having a thorough and comprehensive workup to check your hormone levels.

What are some of the most common causes of hormonal imbalance? Toxins, of all types and sizes:

- Stress
- Obesity
- Poor sleep
- Poor detox
- Dysbiosis due to something like candida overgrowth
- SIBO
- Nutritional insufficiency
- Thyroid dysfunction
- Genetics

- Insulin resistance
- Standard American Diet (SAD)
- Eating disorders
- Alcohol
- Tobacco
- Food sensitivities
- Xenoestrogens
- Environmental Toxins
- Medications [OCP (oral contraceptives)]

Xenoestrogens

Xenoestrogens are a **particularly nasty type of toxin** because they are any foreign substance that mimics the effects of estrogen or promotes its production. They are close enough in molecular structure to estrogen that they can bind to estrogen receptor sites with potentially hazardous outcomes. They have been introduced into our environment for roughly the last 70 years. What are some examples?

Ethinylestradiol (combined oral contraceptive pill)

Chlorine

Food:

- Erythrosine & Phenosulfothiazine (red dyes for food)
- Butylated hydroxyanisole / BHA (food preservative)

Insecticides:

- Atrazine (weed killer)
- DDT, Dieldrin, Endosulfan, Heptachlor, Lindane, Methoxychlor

Skincare:

- 4-Methylbenzylidene camphor (4-MBC) (sunscreen)
- Benzophenone (sunscreen lotions)
- Parabens (commonly used as a preservatives)

Industrial Products and Plastics:

- Plasticizers such as phthalates, bisphenol A, DEHP (plasticizer for PVC)
- Polybrominated biphenyl ethers (PBDEs) (flame retardants used in plastics, foams, building materials, electronics, furnishings, motor vehicles)
- Polychlorinated biphenyls (PCBs)

Building Supplies:

- Pentachlorophenol (wood preservative)
- Polychlorinated biphenyls (PCBs) (in electrical oils, lubricants, adhesives, paints)

According to the Environmental Working Group (ewg.org), women are exposed to 168 different chemicals on their faces every day.[134] And remember there are estrogen receptors in the central nervous system (CNS), blood vessels, lungs, heart, kidneys, uterus, breasts, liver, gut, ovaries, bladder, and bones… which means imbalances in estrogen could have an effect on any of these parts of the body.

What are some of the most common imbalances we see?

- Early menarche (precocious puberty)
- Estrogen dominance (by far and away the most common I see in my practice)
- Luteal phase dysfunction
- Fluctuations in hormone levels
- Hormonal insufficiencies
- Sub-optimal hormone metabolism

Early Menarche and Precocious Puberty

Typically this occurs when a girl's physical signs of sexual maturity develop too soon, including:

- Breast development before age 8
- Menstrual cycle before age 10
- A growth spurt before age 8

Precocious puberty can also occur in boys before the age of 9, and the signs can include:

- Enlargement of the testicles or penis
- Rapid height growth (a growth spurt)

Here is the craziest part: This is what Stanford Health says about precocious puberty:

> It may be caused by tumors or growths on the ovaries, adrenal glands, pituitary gland, or brain. Other causes

may include central nervous system problems, family history of the disease, or certain rare genetic syndromes. In many cases, no cause can be found for the disorder.[135]

Get the func out! This is an example of where people can lose their trust in "science." We just listed so many substances that children are exposed to regularly that could contribute to this condition, but according to one of the most trusted resources in medicine, there is no mention of any of them. So, what is more common, a rare genetic disorder or our toxic environment?

It is traditional medicine's default answer—that these conditions are rapidly on the rise, are known to be influenced by our environment, and are just happening, and "we don't know why." Ever met a child who played with plastic toys or drank from a plastic bottle? Or who applied sunscreen to protect their skin from the sun? Or ate nonorganic fruits and vegetables?

Although I don't know of any direct causation studies that show these toxins being the cause, I think one of the issues is that we are always trying to find "one specific cause." When it comes to toxins, it is rarely just one toxin that is the problem: it is our toxic load, our bucket overflowing, because we are inundated by them. So when it comes to precocious puberty there is not much you can do once it has started, but you can definitely reduce toxic accumulation by cleaning up your environment and getting the func out of your child's body. Did you know that the average newborn has over 200 chemicals in their cord blood?[136]

Estrogen Dominance

This is the most common undiagnosed issue I see with pre-menopausal women in my practice. Estrogen dominance is the condition of increased estrogen levels relative to progesterone levels in the body. Estrogen dominance may be the result of overproduction of estrogen by the body, changes in estrogen metabolism and excretion, or an imbalance in the estrogen to progesterone ratio—and there is no consensus on what the correct ratio is, yet it likely varies significantly between women and can change over time. Estrogen and progesterone levels can be, and still usually are, within normal range. In my practice over half of women, maybe even three in four, during their reproductive years, have estrogen dominance. When we order testing, I tell my patients that it is most likely your numbers will come back in the normal range, but I like to look at exactly where in the normal range, and more importantly—what are your symptoms?

Remember symptoms of estrogen dominance can be:

- PMS
- Weight gain (particularly in hips, midsection, thighs)
- Fibrocystic breasts
- Fibroids
- Endometriosis
- Abnormal menstruation
- Fatigue
- Hair Loss
- Cold/Hands Feet
- Reduced sex drive
- Depression
- Anxiety
- Bloating
- Infertility
- Breast tenderness
- Mood swings
- Brain fog/Memory loss
- Insomnia

If you're diagnosed with estrogen dominance but your estrogen is not even high, what else could be going on? What about xenoestrogens? What if bucket has been getting filled with toxins that mimic the effect of estrogen? In this case, your estrogen levels are normal, but your body thinks they are 10 times higher because of all the toxic effects. Difficult to prove, but I refuse to give up on my patients and be a traditional doctor who says, "I have no idea because the pharmaceutical industry (otherwise known as medical school in my opinion) didn't teach me how to help you." A common way I have been able to diagnose estrogen dominance is progesterone levels during the luteal phase (in the second half of the cycle).

Let's look at some "normal" hormone numbers:

	Follicular Phase	Ovulatory Phase (can be called mid cycle peak)	Luteal Phase
FSH	2.5-10.2 mIU/mL	3.1-17.7 mIU/mL	1.5-9.1 mIU/mL
LH	1.9-12.5 mIU/mL	8.7- 76.3 mIU/mL	0.5-16.9 mIU/mL
Estradiol	19-144 pg/ml	64-357 pg/ml	56- 214 pg/ml
Progesterone	< 1.0 ng/ml		2.6 - 21.5 ng/ml

The two most important things to understand about these numbers is: look at the ranges—they're all over the place! And as we discussed earlier, normal numbers likely vary significantly between women and can change over the course of time. I can't even count the number of women who have come through my office and said, "Yes, my doctor checked my hormones and said they were all normal," but the woman has half of the symptoms of estrogen dominance. My response to this? Get the func out of here! With those vast ranges of normal, the odds of falling outside of them is slim to none.

My first question always is, what phase of your cycle were you in when you tested? Most of the time the patient responds, "I don't know, my doctor didn't advise me when to get tested." When looking for estrogen dominance, it is critical to be tested in the middle of the luteal phase, somewhere between days 19 to 23; I usually recommend day 21. At any other point of the cycle, the progesterone will be zero or close to zero, and this is totally normal. But if your progesterone is 4 ng/ml on day 21 and you have symptoms, I will be recommending a treatment plan for estrogen dominance. So remember, it is of utmost importance to know where you are in your cycle to try to diagnose estrogen dominance.

There is debate over what is an optimal level. I like to see somewhere between 10 to 15 ng/ml around day 21 of the cycle. But remember, every woman is different and her normal level may be different; so my advice is to look at the number but to most importantly listen to your symptoms.

Estrogen Metabolites

Another important lab test can be a urine test measuring the metabolites of the different types of estrogen. We learned earlier that the way estrogen is metabolized can play a major role in influencing disease. The most common one I use looks at the ratio of 2/16 hydroxyestrogens. This number is calculated by dividing the levels of 2-hydroxyestrone and 2-hydroxyestradiol (2-OHE1 + 2-OHE2) and 16α-hydroxyestrone (16α-OH E1). Per the Genova diagnostics website: Estrogen metabolism and the ratio of 2-hydroxyestrogens to 16α-hydroxyestrone has been used to identify patients at risk for cancer and other hormone-related diseases in both men and women. Relative increases in levels of the 2-hydroxylation pathway metabolites are associated with decreased risk.[137,138,139,140,141,142]

Other Hormone Testing

I would like to make a comment on saliva and DUTCH testing for hormones. For many people familiar with the Functional Medicine world, they have done or heard of these tests. I have never ordered one, but I have had many patients come in with the results. Sometimes they are accurate, but most of the time they're not. Urine testing has the fewest clinical validation studies, and can give you a result that is a combination of both the endocrine gland production and peripheral production of conjugated hormones and metabolites. Saliva testing is a measure of unbound, free, active hormone. These hormone levels are extremely low and therefore difficult to measure. Some hormones, like cortisol, DHEA, and estrogens, can come very close to blood levels. Others, like progesterone, do not. And when it comes to the female hormones, the most important number I look at is progesterone. My advice is to forget these tests and check your serum levels, unless you are looking at estrogen metabolites. Some other tips for testing include doing the testing the same way each time (e.g., fasting first thing in the morning on the same day of the cycle).

Premenstrual Syndrome (PMS)

PMS is a combination of physical and emotional symptoms (i.e., nervous tension, mood swings, irritability, anxiety, cramping, bloating, pain, depression, insomnia, and breast tenderness) that happen during the luteal phase (second half of the cycle) and usually subside two days after a new period starts. This likely occurs because estrogen and progesterone levels fall drastically, if pregnancy doesn't occur and the symptoms go away after the body starts making estrogen again at the start of the period.

Over 90% of women have reported PMS symptoms.[143] Just like hormone levels, symptoms can vary dramatically. The average length is about 6 days, and they can be very mild or they can be so severe the woman has to miss work or school (this is called premenstrual dysphoric disorder (PMDD). PMS is more likely in women who have a history of depression or high levels of stress.[144,145] There is no test to diagnose PMS; the diagnosis is made based on symptoms. Half of women with PMS also have another condition like depression, anxiety, chronic fatigue, IBS, or bladder pain syndrome.[146]

This brings up the whole point of Functional medicine. In my practice, I do not worry so much about what the diagnosis is, but what the imbalances are. Because when the body is imbalanced, the symptoms will normally show up in more than one area. One specific diet that was found to be helpful is a low-fat vegetarian diet; it was found to increase sex hormone binding globulin (SHBG), which lowers the free-circulating hormone levels.[147] Increasing your fiber intake also helps you eliminate estrogen by decreasing its reuptake.

There are some other common diagnoses someone could have like dysmenorrhea (cramps), menorrhagia (heavy periods), amenorrhea (no periods), and PCOS (multiple cysts in the ovaries, discussed briefly in the last chapter), for which I would recommend a similar approach. PCOS is particularly interesting, as high sugar intake causing elevated insulin is the most likely underlying cause. Elevated insulin leads to improper FSH and LH secretion, which causes more androgens to be made. When a woman has PCOS, ovulation does not occur, and estrogens are not opposed by progesterone, causing estrogen excess. Elevated insulin also leads to decreased sex hormone-binding globulin (SHBG) which leads to an increase in free testosterone. The goal of treatment is the same: Identify and treat imbalances in the body.

Let's look at some of my favorite treatment options. A reminder, the quality of the supplement is a huge determining factor in whether it will be effective. How long treatment can take depends on the individual and their history, and you should have a trusted practitioner that will help guide you along the way.

	Function	Daily Dose	Goal of Treatment
Bioidentical Progesterone Replacement	• Replace a hormone which is deficient • Down-regulates estrogen receptors • Affects DNA transcription, cellular adhesion • Increases cellular differentiation • Involved in initiation of ovulation • Inhibits uterine activity • Induction of enzymes important in estrogen metabolism	• 50 - 200mg capsule at night one hour before bed on days 14 to 28 of your cycle • If period starts early stop progesterone, if doesn't start, stop on day 28 • My preferred route is oral capsules. Many practitioners use cream, which I have found to be ineffective • Do not buy off the Internet without doctor's prescription	• All perimenopausal women need progesterone • Decreases PMS symptoms • Protects against uterine and breast cancer, osteoporosis, fibrocystic disease, ovarian cysts, and coronary artery disease • Progesterone opens up the liver to help in detox • Do not use progestins, which are synthetic forms of the body's naturally occurring hormone progesterone; when you see studies of progesterone linked to cancers, it is synthetic hormones

	Function	Daily Dose	Goal of Treatment
Chasteberry (Vitex)	• Comes from a shrub that makes a peppery fruit • Likely affects dopamine, acetylcholine and opioid receptors.	20 - 40mg	• Decrease irregularities of the menstrual cycle and symptoms of PMS • Should NOT be used In patients with fibroids, endometriosis, or high breast cancer risk, because it can have pro-estrogenic effects[148]
Calcium	Deficiency in PMS[149]	500 - 1200mg for 2-3 cycles	Decrease PMS symptoms (cramps, bloating, food cravings)
Vitamin B6	• Anti-inflammatory • Helps glucose regulation • Cofactor for neurotransmitter synthesis including serotonin, dopamine, epinephrine and norepinephrine	50 - 100mg	Decrease anxiety, stabilize sugar, decreases inflammation
Magnesium	Cofactor for neurotransmitter synthesis including serotonin and dopamine Has vasomotor effects	450mg of magnesium citrate at night is my preferred choice	Reduce PMS symptoms
Vitamin D	Deficiency in PMS[150]	Dose to levels, wants levels to be between 60-100 ng/mL	Decrease PMS symptoms

Even moderate alcohol consumption is linked to both increases in estrogen and decreases in progesterone.[151] There are also supplements to support the proper detox of estrogen.

Glutathione (I only use liposomal)	One TSP first thing in the morning (I prefer the Readisorb brand)
N Acetyl Cysteine (Is a precursor to making glutathione, I prefer glutathione)	600 - 1,200mg daily
Indole 3 carbinol	200 - 400mg daily
Vitamin C	1000 - 3000mg daily
EPA/DHA (fish oil)	1000 - 4000 mg daily

End of Reproductive Years

Let's take a look at a few more things women experience hormonally over the course of their lifetime.

Perimenopause

Considered the transition phase between the end of reproductive years and menopause (the end of fertility), perimenopause is thought to be due to a rapid decline in estrogen. It can last 4 to 8 years and usually starts in the 40s, sometimes in the 30s. A woman has a set number of oocytes and that number decreases as she gets older; during perimenopause the decrease accelerates. Risks for perimenopause include: smoking, cancer treatment, hysterectomy, autoimmune issues, and toxins. Symptoms can include hot flashes, night sweats, headaches, anxiety, nausea, and changes in heart rate. A very interesting discovery is that hot flashes are not triggered based on estrogen levels but on adrenaline. Yes, your adrenals play a role in hot flashes (a.k.a. stress and unresolved trauma).[152] What are some supplements that could help with perimenopause?

Perimenopause		Daily Dose	Goal of Treatment
Black Cohosh	• Has some anti-estrogenic properties • Antioxidant • Has some activity against breast cancer cell proliferation[153]	20mg twice daily	• Can reduce menopausal symptoms and hot flash frequency • It can have same effect as low-dose hormonal therapy for relieving menopausal symptoms • Not all studies support its effectiveness[154]
Soy	• Can be effective due to high levels of isoflavones • Can act as selective estrogen receptor modulators (increase good estrogen decrease bad estrogen)	Only eat Non-GMO organic forms of soy	May slow bone loss, improve depression, cognition, and have cardiovascular benefits
Bioidentical Progesterone Replacement	• Replace a hormone which is deficient • Down-regulates estrogen receptors • Affects DNA transcription, cellular adhesion • Increases cellular differentiation • Involved in initiation of ovulation • Inhibits uterine activity • Induction of enzymes important in estrogen metabolism	My preferred dosing is 100mg capsule twice daily; some people have success with days 14 to 28 of period, if periods are relatively regular—please work with an experienced practitioner because it can vary	See page 72

Menopause

Just like the female reproductive hormone cycle, we will end with menopause. Menopause is signaled by 12 months since last menstruation. It most commonly occurs between the mid-40s and mid-50s. Symptoms can include: hot flashes, sleep disturbances, loss of bladder control, vaginal dryness, irritability, depression, weight gain, and stiff muscles and joints. It does not sound fun and I feel a great compassionate for women going through it. While not all women get menopause symptoms, one study reported that 85% of women have experienced symptoms related to menopause.[155] What's more interesting is that 73% of women don't attempt any treatment for their symptoms.[156]

I think the most important part of the menopause discussion is that is a natural biological process. By talking to different Functional Medicine doctors or traditional doctors, you will hear different opinions on whether hormone replacement therapy (HRT) is appropriate. My least favorite thing are hormone clinics where everybody walking through the door gets put on hormones. These clinics frequently label themselves as Functional Medicine, but just prescribing hormones is not Functional Medicine. The more humane method is to base treatments on the severity of symptoms and what the patient wants, so I don't push hormone replacement on anyone who is not interested in it.

I really like the book *Healthy Aging* by Neal Rozier, MD, as a resource about the pros and cons of HRT. I would argue it is not for everyone, especially not if there is history of brain tumor, active breast cancer, family history of breast cancer, any kind of clotting disorder or family history of clotting disorder, unaddressed vaginal bleeding, liver disease, genetic issues, or someone who tried HRT and had a negative reaction.

Some of the main health risks for women of menopausal age include heart disease, osteoporosis, and cognitive decline. So the primary argument for HRT is that it may protect a woman's heart, but the data can vary depending on who you believe. If it is something you choose to do, then the earlier the better.[157] If a woman has a high risk of cardiac disease and low risk of cancer, HRT may be a good option.

Regarding the risk of osteoporosis, 1 in 3 women world-wide over the age of 50 will experience osteoporotic fractures. During menopause, bone breakdown is increased, leading to more osteoporosis. HRT slows down the breakdown of bone and can help prevent osteoporosis. Loss of hormones may also contribute to cognitive decline, so HRT may also help prevent it. There is heated debate over HRT for menopause. Although I have helped patients with this, it is not my specialty. If you are going to do it, I do recommend using estrogen, progesterone, and testosterone that is based on your lab work. Most importantly, find a practitioner that you trust: one who has proven experience, and will go over the pluses and minuses of it for you specifically.

CHAPTER 5

Male Hormones

Now a subject near and dear to my heart, testosterone. It is thought of as "the male hormone," but women produce it and also experience symptoms if they don't have enough. Testosterone production is controlled by the pituitary gland and hypothalamus in your brain, just like thyroid, cortisol, and the female reproductive hormones. In men, most of the production of testosterone comes from the testes; in women it is produced in the ovaries and adrenal glands.

Why is testosterone so great? It is anabolic, which means it makes things grow! It regulates sex drive (libido), bone mass, fat distribution, muscle mass and strength, and the production of red blood cells and sperm. A man's testosterone level starts to decline after the age of 30 (it can even start at 25) and continues to decrease by about 1 percent a year for the rest of his life. Almost 40% of men age 45 and older have low testosterone. Only 1% to 2% of testosterone circulates in blood as unbound "free" testosterone, but this fraction exhibits the most potent biological activity.

Again the major difference we have between the traditional medical world and the functional medicine world is the ranges, and therefore what we each consider normal. We will get in detail on lab testing soon.

First, let's talk a little bit about how testosterone is

made and what it does. Did you know that 95% of testosterone is made in Leydig cells, which are in the testes? The rest comes from the adrenal glands, which make DHEA and androstenedione, which are precursors to testosterone. Testosterone, just like other hormones we have discussed, is made from cholesterol. The signal to produce testosterone starts in the brain from a hormone called GnRH, which is made by the hypothalamus; it is secreted in pulses that tell your pituitary gland to make LH and FSH, which are what travel down and stimulate the testes to make testosterone. FSH stimulates Sertoli cells to help sperm production and maturation, and LH stimulates Leydig cells to make testosterone. What's interesting is that this pathway operates via a negative feedback loop. When testosterone is made, it shuts down LH, FSH and GnRH production. Some other major players in the testosterone pathway include:

DHT (Dihydrotestosterone)

About 10% of testosterone produced daily is converted into DHT. DHT is much more powerful than testosterone; it is thought to have similar effects to T3 from your thyroid. DHT is what is thought to initiate puberty and development of reproductive organs, promotes expression of male sexual behavior, and causes the prostate to grow (a commonly prescribed medicine called finasteride blocks DHT production and is used for benign prostate hypertrophy). DHT has many beneficial effects but take note: too much DHT has been found in men with male pattern baldness.[158]

Estrogen

A very interesting part of the testosterone loop is estrogen. A small amount of circulating testosterone is converted to estradiol, the active form of estrogen, via an enzyme called 5 alpha reductase. Estradiol has some important functions in men, but just like women, you don't want too much. Estrogen in men can improve cognitive function, and helps prevent bone loss and the loss of blood sugar control, while too much estrogen can contribute to BPH. One of the greatest risks for excess estradiol is obesity, as fat cells make estrogen.

DHEA

A lot of controversy surrounds DHEA. It does not require a prescription, is made as a supplement, and was marketed as the fountain of youth. Produced in the adrenal glands, it is thought to be converted into testosterone (this is how it was marketed), but studies have found that it is not converted in the blood in men and very little in women. DHEA is thought to have its own receptors that give it some benefit;[159] specifically, DHEA has been found to have positive effects on cardiovascular health.[160] Most people take it to increase testosterone but it is not an effective treatment for testosterone production.

What are some of the ways testosterone affects the body?

Cognitive Function

Some studies have shown cognitive improvement from testosterone replacement.[161] There are androgen receptors all over the brain, so when free testosterone circulates, it can bind and work on these receptors. DHT, as the more potent hormone, binds the androgen receptors in the brain with a greater affinity than testosterone.[162]

Muscle

Testosterone increases muscle mass by increasing muscle protein synthesis[163] and inhibiting protein breakdown.[164] Athletes discovered that certain derivatives of testosterone had greater ability at this than others (DHT is not one of these). Think anabolic steroids, think baseball players in the late 1990s and 2000s. Look at Barry Bonds (notably a central figure in baseball's steroids scandal) when he started his career on the Pirates and when he ended it on the Giants.

Fat

Testosterone inhibits adipocytes, the cells that make fat grow, and it stimulates lipolysis (fat breakdown) by increasing the number of lipolytic receptors.[165]

Mitochondria

The powerhouse of our cells! Mitochondria are where we produce energy. Testosterone stimulates glucose utilization and ATP production,[166] and testosterone stimulates specifically mitochondrial cytochrome c oxidase activity in muscle.

Immune System

Testosterone is thought to be an immune system modulator,[167] which means it helps regulate inflammatory response. A study in 2021 found that low testosterone was a risk factor for severe COVID-19 infection.[168]

Bone

Testosterone stimulates bone growth and strength, activates osteoblasts, and inhibits osteoclasts. Men with low testosterone were found to have lower bone density and increased risk of fracture.[169] Estrogen also helps bones grow, and remember, testosterone can be converted to estradiol.

Heart

The heart also has androgen receptors. Low testosterone may increase the risk of developing coronary artery disease (CAD), metabolic syndrome, and type 2 diabetes.[170] Men with low testosterone treated with HRT had decreased body weight, leptin, and insulin levels.[171] There is a protein called lipoprotein (LP a) which is an independent risk factor for heart disease; testosterone therapy has been shown to decrease Lp a by over 30%.[172]

So in theory, having low testosterone could make you feel slower, with brain fog, poor memory, low energy, low athletic endurance, increased weight, higher body fat, weak bones, increased fractures, higher blood sugar and higher cholesterol, increasing your risk of heart disease. Yikes. And we saw that having low testosterone is actually very common.

So What Lowers Testosterone?

Aging

SHBG (sex hormone binding globulin) levels rise with age, causing free testosterone levels to fall.[173] Remember, SHBG is what modulates how many androgens are available to your tissues. Testosterone that is bound to SHBG is inactive; it factors into one's total testosterone value, but it is free testosterone that binds to receptors. If the levels of SHBG are higher, more testosterone will be bound and less will be available to work on tissues.

The number of Leydig cells decreases after men turn 20 years old.[174] They begin life with 700 million Leydig cells and lose six million of those cells yearly after their twentieth birthday.[175] And remember, these are the cells that make 95% of testosterone. GnRH and LH also decrease as we age, shutting down the signal to make testosterone.

Stress (Cortisol)

The stress hormone, cortisol, blocks an enzyme called 17 alpha hydroxylase, which is part of pathway that converts cholesterol into eventually testosterone.

Obesity

Obese teen boys have up to 50 percent less testosterone than lean boys.[176] Obesity increases inflammation, which can be seen as high IL-6 levels, which shuts down Leydig and Sertoli cell function.[177] Low testosterone also makes it more likely that you will be obese. So it's a which-came-first thing? The chicken or the egg? The low testosterone-causing obesity or obesity causing low testosterone? From a Functional Medicine standpoint, it doesn't really matter; we need to address all root causes.

Insulin

Insulin inhibits another enzyme called 17,20 lyase, which prevents testosterone production and stimulates testosterone metabolism to estradiol. Remember, insulin is one of the two hormones you don't want too much of.

Alcohol and Opiates

Alcohol suppresses testosterone production from the testes and increases aromatase activity; aromatase is what causes testosterone to be converted to estradiol. (Other factors that increase aromatase are: zinc deficiency, insulin, obesity, cortisol, and toxins like BPA.) Opioid use induces severe low testosterone.[178]

Lack of Sleep

One of our favorite factors that is so commonly overlooked, sleep. We spend so much time talking about foods, viruses, toxins, and hormones as underlying causes for disease, but we tend to forget that without adequate sleep, nothing functions well. One study limited men to 5 hours of sleep per night, and found a daily decreased testosterone level between 10% and 15% lower.[179]

Toxins

Phthalates and Bisphenol A (from plastics), heavy metals like lead and mercury (from air and food), and PBDE (flame retardant in furniture) lower testosterone levels in utero, before you're even born, and then throughout life.[180,181]

Who is not at risk for low testosterone? Seems like the majority of men in our current environment are at risk. If you're a man reading this, or thinking of your significant other, you probably want to know, *how do we find out if testosterone is low?* Here are the lab tests that I will order.

Serum Testing	Reference Range	Comments
Total Testosterone	250 - 1100 ng/dl	• Test first thing in the morning • Look at that range! • What is optimal? Most say between 650 - 1100 ng/dl, but it depends on the individual
Free Testosterone	35 - 155 pg/mL	• Arguably the more important number, as it indicates how much T is available to bind to receptors • Total and Free T should be looked at together • Too much causes fluid retention, acne, increased appetite and weight gain, increased muscle mass, mood swings
PSA	< 4 ng/mL	• Must be monitored if on testosterone replacement • PSA will usually rise when starting testosterone replacement
% Free PSA (if PSA is elevated)	>25 % (calc)	• % free PSA is used to increase the specificity of total PSA when PSA levels are between 4 - 10 and to prevent unnecessary biopsy • A low % indicates increased cancer risk
LH	1.5 - 9.3 mIU/mL	• Stimulates testosterone production • Will be suppressed if on T replacement
FSH	1.6 - 8.0 mIU/mL	• Stimulates sperm production and maturation • Will be suppressed if on T replacement

Serum Testing	Reference Range	Comments
SHBG	Varies by age 18 - 55 Years; 17 - 124 nmol/L	• SHBG carries testosterone, DHT, estradiol throughout your bloodstream • In general, a low reading will mean more free hormones available and a high reading would mean less hormones available
Estradiol	≤39 pg/mL	• Elevates when aromatase activity is increased, symptoms of too much could be erectile dysfunction (ED) and breast growth
DHT	12 - 65 ng/dL	• Too much is associated with male pattern baldness, acne, prostate growth • Levels within range can improve blood sugar, memory, sexual function, decreased coronary artery disease
DHEA	Varies by age 31 - 40 years; 106 - 464 mcg/dL 61 - 70 Years; 24 - 244 mcg/dL	• Does not convert to testosterone in blood
Ferritin	Varies by age 19 - 59 years; 38 - 380 ng/mL	• A marker of how much iron is stored; levels can decrease when on testosterone replacement
CBC	Focus is on Hemoglobin and Hematocrit	• Watch out for elevated Hgb and Hct when on testosterone replacement

*Just like with the female hormones, I am not a fan of saliva or urine testing. There are labs with good marketing that will make these seem better, but I have always used blood testing. It doesn't have the controversy the others do and it also is usually covered by insurance.

These ranges are all over the place!!! So what is "normal?" I don't think we know for sure; I think it varies from person to person. One man may feel OK with a free T of 45 pg/mL whereas another man could have the symptoms of low testosterone at a free T of 60 pg/mL. It is of the utmost importance to find a practitioner who has experience in working with men with low testosterone.

If you're a man, when should you consider low testosterone?

- Age 25 or older
- Low sex drive
- Difficulty with erection
- Low semen volume
- Hair loss
- Fatigue
- Loss of muscle mass
- Increased body fat
- Decreased bone mass
- Mood changes: irritability, depression, lack of focus
- Poor memory and concentration
- Low blood count

Now for why testosterone is near and dear to my heart. I was diagnosed with low testosterone at the age of 35 years old, but I believe it started way before that. The biggest symptom I felt was that I was different than my friends growing up, in that I would work out as much as they did and never could get my body to where I wanted it. I had poor muscle definition, more body fat. Looking back, it could have been due to my lifestyle, binge drinking every weekend and never paying attention to my diet (I ate way too much fast food). But even when my diet got healthier, my body composition didn't change.

An astute doctor and I were talking about my health, and I told her about some of my other symptoms like low sex drive, hair loss, and depression. She said, "I think you have low testosterone."

I laughed in her face. I said, "I'm 35, I don't have low T."

When I humored her and tested, my total testosterone came back at 219 and my free T was 28. As soon as I saw the numbers I had an *agh-ha* moment. Now all the symptoms I thought were just normal for me made sense. It made me feel inadequate and like a failure, but looking at my risk factors (i.e., the alcohol, the diet, the stress, and the high levels of lead I ended up finding in my body), it is not surprising my testosterone was in the tank.

This being the case, I was advised to go on testosterone replacement. I used a bioidentical cream, twice a day for 3 years. It was the best 3 years of my life to date. My mood was good, my libido was high, and finally all the work I was putting in at the gym was paying off, with my body looking the way I thought it always should. I was already in recovery at this point so alcohol was out of my life, and I was deep in the Functional Medicine world so my diet was clean; I was following a Mediterranean diet high in vegetable and fruit intake. About 2 years in, I met Mackenzie and as time went on we knew we wanted to have a family together.

At first, my thought was: *this is going to be great, I'm on the testosterone, I must have great sperm and fertility.* I had honestly never thought about any of the negative side effects testosterone might be having on my body; I felt amazing and when I tested my levels they were perfect. But when I started thinking about having a family, I did some research into testosterone replacement and I was horrified. As it tuns out, testosterone replacement may be the best form of birth control for men on Earth.

I was outraged. *How did the doctor who put me on it never mention it?* More so, I was mad at myself. *How did I not know this?* It is totally embarrassing as physician for me to admit, but years of practicing medicine and recovery have to taught me humility and I am able to acknowledge when I don't know something. My own truth was that I felt so good I chose never to think about side effects. With this new information, I ordered a sperm analysis. *Maybe my body was different?*

My results came back with normal semen levels, but no sperm. I was devastated. What had I done to myself? Luckily Mackenzie was the most supportive partner I have ever had and she kept me going while I was down in the dumps. I immediately stopped the testosterone. Some may be wondering, why did this happen? It is not totally obvious for all of us, including me. Low testosterone is associated with low sperm and low fertility, so why would increasing testosterone stop sperm production?

It comes down to the negative feedback cycle I mentioned earlier in this chapter. When testosterone goes up, LH and FSH go down. No big deal with LH, because it tells my body to make testosterone, but woah, no FSH, means no sperm. Having these signals shut down for 3 years told my body not to make sperm. Simple science that my doctor and I missed. I thank God I never put a man in reproductive age on testosterone replacement without this information.

I immediately became an expert in supporting sperm production (I can gladly say I make lots of sperm again). What helped me the most was a medication called clomiphene. Women with issues with ovulation may be very familiar with this drug, or men who want to boost their testosterone (and sperm) production.

Male Infertility

What are other reasons infertility is on the rise? This is crazy, but did you know that sperm counts among men in North America, Europe, Australia and New Zealand declined more than 59% from 1973 to 2011. What is the one consistent thing during that time period? Our entire environment just gets more and more toxic—our food, our air, our water, our stress—and there is a pretty significant correlation with the timing.

What are some of the key toxins? Organophosphates, solvents, lead and mercury, air pollution, phthalates, and PCBs are associated with reduced sperm concentration,[182,183] reduced motility and morphology. Commonly used drugs have been found to be related to infertility, as well as alcohol (3 drinks daily) and marijuana (a study found it plays a role in disrupting spermatogenesis and sperm function).[184]

Clomiphene

Clomiphene is FDA approved for anovulation in females, but is also frequently used off label in men, the common dose is 50mg daily. The story of my life seems to be make mistakes, fall down, and then get back up. Clomiphene was part of my story of getting back up. Clomiphene, an estrogen receptor modulator, is both pro and anti-estrogenic, which means it turns it on and off. It is a partial agonist of estrogen in the hypothalamus, causing negative-feedback inhibition to increase GnRH production, which increases FSH and LH, which causes testosterone and sperm production (in women not ovulating, this induces ovulation and can lead to twin births). Traditional medicine is amazing in terms of the things they can do to your body.

There is percentage of men who don't ever make sperm again after being on testosterone for an extended time; it is usually related to age, the older the more likely,[185] but naturally my underlying fear was that it would be me. After 6 months, we retested my sperm and I was still shooting blanks. During this time, the other major things I did were: get the heavy metals out of my body, and use supplements that boost sperm production, both of which we will get into soon. I was getting great sleep, being strict with my diet, exercising daily, praying nightly, meditating daily, doing a gratitude list, and in therapy every 2 weeks to talk about my issues. We tested again after one year and I was back! Sperm concentration, volume, motility all WNL (within normal limits)! It was a celebration!

Let's look at some of the supplements I was using and how they work. I did not take all of these but want you to have the full list.

Zinc	30-60mg	Increases testosterone[186]
Tribulus	750mg	Increases testosterone[187]
Fenugreek	600mg	Increases testosterone[188]
Vitamin D	Dose to levels	Increases testosterone[189]
Coenzyme Q10	100 - 300mg	Protects testosterone from toxins. Works as an antioxidant preventing free radical damage[190]
Acetyl L Carnitine	500 - 600mg twice daily	Increases testosterone, LH, FSH. Also acts as antioxidant preventing the attack of toxins on hormones[191]
Vitamin E	400mg	Increases testosterone[192]
Vitamin C	1,000mg	Increases FSH, improves sperm motility, increases testosterone[193]
Aspartic Acid	2,000 - 3,000mg	Likely increases testosterone[194]
Ashwagandha	1,000 - 5,000mg	Increases DHEA and testosterone[195]
Korean Ginseng (Panax Ginseng)	2,000mg daily	Shown to be effective treatment for erectile dysfunction[196]
Maca Root	1,500 - 2,400mg	Increases sexual desire[197]

What a list! Let's just say that when I got off of testosterone and was trying to regain my sperm, I had a very full pill box!

Testosterone Replacement

Most importantly, in my experience, there is not one right way to do testosterone replacement. It is very different for every man and woman. Women on testosterone replacement can feel improved well-being, improved energy, improved strength & endurance, improved body composition, improved bone density, improved sexual function, and increased clitoral sensitivity; they may experience a decrease in visceral fat and maintain muscle mass; and just for skin, it can increase collagen, increase skin thickness, improve texture, decrease in wrinkles, and decrease cellulite.[198]

When it comes to testosterone replacement, we are not talking Barry Bonds; we are shooting for a "normal" level. When I was on T replacement, my levels maintained between 700 and 1,000 ng/dl. I felt great at these levels, but I have worked with men who felt best at the high end or didn't feel good at the high end of normal. Again, it is extremely individualized. Let's also talk briefly about the route of replacement, because there are many different options and each man will find what works best for him. For me it was cream applied twice daily, but other routes (with comments) include:

Injectable: While injectable T is very common in traditional medicine, my main concern is that levels elevate very high after injection and then slowly go down over 1 to 2 weeks. For example, they may rise to 2000 ng/dl the day after injection and then dip back to 200 after 2 weeks. This can be a shock to the body.

Patches: Difficult compliancy (meaning people don't remember to put their patch on when their supposed to).

Troche (Troche are small, hard tablets designed to dissolve slowly over 30 minutes or so when placed under the tongue): Poor absorption leading to a minimal increase in serum testosterone levels.

Topical Gels: Common in traditional medicine, and better results than injection, in my clinical experience.

Oral: Overall I do not recommend this route, as it is toxic to the liver.

Pellets (About the size of a grain of rice, they are implanted under the skin, and are supposed to deliver testosterone slowly for up to 3-6 months at a time): Costly, requiring a surgical procedure every 3-6 months; the absorption is irregular.

Contraindications to Testosterone Replacement

- Active prostate cancer
- Pregnant women or transference to one (if the cream or gel is applied and you snug your partner, it can transfer to them)
- Women who might become pregnant
- Men with fertility issues

Possible Side Effects

- Prostate enlargement
- Hair loss
- Hair growth
- Acne
- Increased libido
- Aggression

- Stops sperm production (can counteract this with other meds like clomiphene)
- Polycythemia, elevated hemoglobin and hematocrit (high blood count)
- Gynecomastia (breast growth; I had one patient in his fifties
- stop T replacement because of this)
- Fluid retention and edema
- Decreased testicle size (usually comes back after stopping treatment)
- Teratogenic (causing birth defects)
- Sleep apnea

The thing you will hear the most from the traditional standpoint is that testosterone replacement causes prostate cancer; however, there is no evidence that testosterone replacement therapy is an independent risk factor for development of prostate cancer.[199]

What Should You Do If You Have Low Testosterone?

As we have learned, the process of optimizing testosterone levels is different for everyone. For many men I work with, they say the same thing I said, that being on testosterone replacement was the best they have ever felt. I have met men who swear by injections, cream, gel, and pellets; I have not seen a way to predict which option will be best for you.

For someone who has never been on hormone replacement, I would start with a bioidentical cream applied twice daily. I also work with men who start with just supplements or just clomiphene, or both, and they are happy with the results. The most important steps are to find a practitioner that you trust who has experience with hormone replacement, that is not running a hormone clinic (putting everyone who walks through the door on hormones), and that willingly listens to your symptoms, tests your levels, and adjusts your plan based on how you are responding to treatment.

There are seven morals to my personal hormone replacement story shared in this chapter. First, nothing comes without side effects (for example side effects of clomiphene include abdominal issues, headache, high triglycerides, and blood clotting). Second, make sure your doctor explains all potential treatments thoroughly. Third, don't give up, and get back up when you fall down. Fourth, always focus on your mental, emotional, spiritual health. Fifth, don't be afraid to admit when you're wrong. Sixth, traditional medicine can be great and alternative medicine can be great. And the lucky seventh, don't ever give up.

CHAPTER 6

Detox

What is detox? If you get on social media and start following your favorite Instagram influencers, you can become quickly convinced that you need to buy their special blend of detox supplements. But do you really need them? Are you toxic?

Just like I think we are all a little bit crazy and need to work on that, I believe we are all a little toxic, but do all of us need to work on that? My answer differs from your favorite influencer: *it depends…what are your symptoms? And what are your bodies toxic levels?* Just like with hormones or gut health, I do not think everyone has an issue and would benefit from treatment simply because they are breathing; I like to rely on the testing and the person's story. Mind you, some testing is better than others, some toxins are easier to identify than others. Let's discuss how to approach toxins.

There are many different approaches practitioners in the Functional Medicine world take, so what you hear from me might be different than what you've learned so far from other physicians and practitioners. I do not believe my way is the only right way. In my own practice, I'm always trying to improve and adjust my treatment plans. Yet we've had a lot of success with detox, and I've also seen a lot of things that *don't* work, so I do want to share my experience to help clarify and simplify what can be an overwhelming concept. I'm excited for you and hope this will be an important piece of your healing journey.

* * *

As you learned in the Introduction, toxins are substances that can cause injury or death, and they can come from living organisms like bacteria or fungi (endotoxins), or they can enter the body from our environment (exotoxins). An interesting fact in my own experience of researching this subject is that a lot of the data seems to disappear or be very difficult to put a finger on. Sometimes articles get published and shortly thereafter, you can't find them. In 2009, 85,000 chemicals were registered for commercial use, but less than ten percent of them had gone through basic testing, looking at things like cancer risk or effects on hormones, immunity, development, or neurological effect.[200] As more and more toxins were introduced into our environment, while the effects on the human population were not considered, it appears the focus was on profits over people. And as more people became sick and demanded answers, we now have independent resources like the Environmental Working Group to provide us with a considerable amount of the data people are searching for.

In the Introduction, I illustrated how toxic a common morning routine can be for the average person. Remember, we're exposed to toxins from food, cleaning products, mattresses, cell phones, plastic food containers, water bottles, air fresheners, fabric softeners, deodorants, dry cleaning, bug sprays, and sunscreen, just to name a few. The most important difference between looking at toxicity from the Functional Medicine standpoint rather than from the traditional medical view is *total toxic burden*. In other words, using the metaphor, "How full is your bucket?" It is most likely that not just your preferred air freshener or fabric softener will make you sick, but it's the cumulative toxin load beginning in utero that over time can cause problems.

Before we dive into the specific toxins, I want to explain what detox is.

Detox

As a great Functional Medicine doctor, Dr. Robert Roundtree, taught me: we are what we eat, drink, breathe, touch, and can't eliminate. (I would add to that, we are also what we think and feel). Detox is our ability to eliminate all the different invaders to which we are exposed. We are all being exposed, but not all of us get sick. Why? I think the number one reason is luck, but reasons someone might not detox well or just be more susceptible to toxins are:

- ongoing toxin exposure
- nutrient deficiencies
- Standard American Diet (SAD)
- stress
- trauma
- dysbiosis or SIBO
- genetics

Most of us think of detox as being just our liver, but other systems that are important to detox are our lymphatics, gut, kidneys, skin, and lungs.

Let's take an example of a toxin like lead, found in paint on walls in older homes. Many people paint over their lead-painted walls and let's say while you are doing this your skin is rubbing against the wall. One of the first lines of defense is your skin. As a barrier, your skin is doing its best to prevent a toxin from entering your body. (The skin as a further potential detox organ is a debatable subject.) An alternative medicine practitioner could tell you acne, blackheads, pimples, and boils usually appear when the liver and kidneys can't get rid of toxins, so they send fat soluble toxins through the oil-secreting glands in your skin to push them out, which creates breakouts. Your traditional dermatologist will likely tell you this is wrong, that the skin has nothing to do with detox, and that the only thing you can do to protect your skin is moisturize and apply sunscreen (a known toxin).

I don't completely agree with either of these views, and just as with most things between the Functional and traditional world, I fall somewhere in-between. From the traditional standpoint, I agree that the skin does not have detox-specific mechanisms like the liver or kidneys do; however your skin does have Langerhan Cells, which are part of your innate immunity that trap toxins breaching the skin barrier. From the Functional standpoint, I agree that sweating is one of the best ways to detox. This insight is based on the most simple fact about detox: toxins are fat soluble, and detox makes them water soluble. In the process, you pee, poop, and sweat them out.

Gut

From all the painting you did, you are feeling dehydrated, so you drink a cup of water, and now the lead from your drinking water is trying to enter through your gut. The most important job of the gut, as covered in *Unfunc Your Gut*, is that it's also a barrier. So if you unfunc'ed your gut and it's not leaky, it will stop the lead from coming in. But what if you haven't unfunc'ed your gut and your gut is leaky? Yes, the lead can cross the gut barrier and get into you blood stream. Now it's free to move around and cause damage. Luckily, you have your liver working for you, and before the toxin can go wreak havoc on your body, the blood stream carries whatever crosses over from the outside environment across your gut to the liver.

The Liver and Gallbladder

The liver sits in the right upper quadrant of your abdomen, weighs about 3 pounds, and may have over 500 functions! But to keep it simple, we're going to focus on its detox function. The liver's job is to maintain metabolic homeostasis (keep things balanced), which includes the processing of amino acids, carbohydrates, fats, vitamins, and minerals coming in from the gut; the liver also removes microbes and toxins, then excretes them through bile. Bile is a thick and sticky, yellow-green fluid produced by the liver and stored in the gallbladder; it helps your body break down fats, absorb vitamins, and remove toxins. The liver produces about 800 to 1,000 mL (27 to 34 fluid ounces) of bile each day;[201] and the gallbladder usually can hold about 30 to 80 mL (about 1 to 2.7 fluid ounces) of fluid, so that leaves roughly 770 to 920 mL (26 to 31 oz.) of bile that flows into your small intestine daily for excretion. Eating fatty foods stimulates the gallbladder to contract and release bile to aid in the breakdown of fat in the small intestine. The smaller fat droplets are easier for the pancreatic enzymes to break down or digest. The bile salts also help the cells in the bowel to absorb fats.

The cells in your liver (hepatocytes) are fed by blood coming from your gut on one side, filtered, pulling toxins out and excreting them via bile flow on the other side. This is where Phase I and Phase II detox happen.

Phase I and Phase II Metabolism (Detox)

Detox is the process by which we make toxins that are fat soluble (and easily stored in our bodies) water soluble so they can be excreted. Phase I are a group of reactions which create a more water-soluble metabolite, which is still active and toxic, called a *reactive oxygen intermediate*, a type of oxidation that can

LIVER DETOXIFICATION PATHWAYS

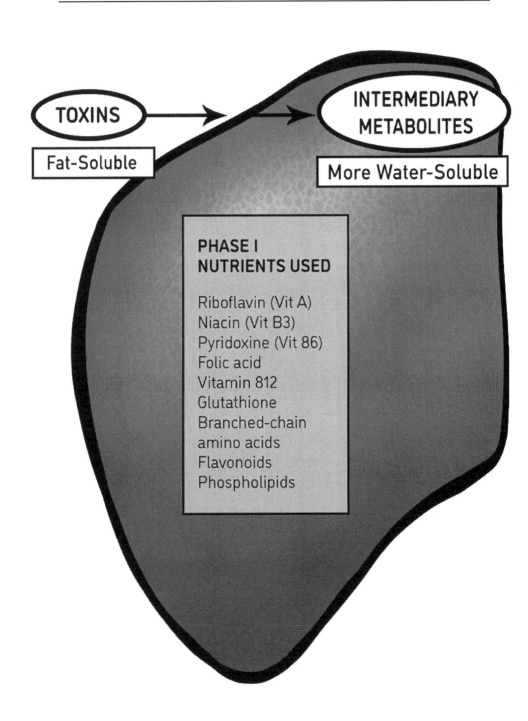

TOXINS

Fat-Soluble

INTERMEDIARY METABOLITES

More Water-Soluble

PHASE I NUTRIENTS USED

Riboflavin (Vit A)
Niacin (Vit B3)
Pyridoxine (Vit 86)
Folic acid
Vitamin 812
Glutathione
Branched-chain amino acids
Flavonoids
Phospholipids

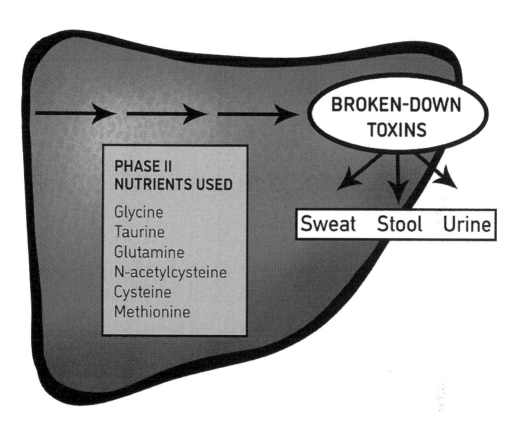

Intermediary Metabolites Can Become Free Radicals, Which Anti-Oxidants Can Protect Against

- Carotenes (Vit A)
- Ascorbic acid (Vit C)
- Tocopherols (Vit E)
- Selenium
- Copper
- Zinc
- Manganese

- Coenzyme Q10
- Thiols
- Bioflavonoids
- Silymarin
- Pycnogenol
- Phospholipids

cause secondary tissue damage. The reactive oxygen intermediate can be neutralized by antioxidants, but if not, the still potentially toxic substance is metabolized by Phase II metabolism. (The pharmaceutical industry uses this to their advantage and makes drugs that need to be metabolized by Phase I to become active.) The different types of reactions which happen in Phase I and Phase II are also dependent on different vitamins and minerals to function and what's more, a number of antioxidants are an important part of this process (see Figure 1).

	Types of Reactions	Nutrients Used
Phase I	Oxidation (most common) Reduction Hydrolysis	Vitamin A Niacin (B3) Pyridoxine (B6) Folic Acid (B9) Cobalamin (B12) Glutathione Branched Chain Amino Acids Flavonoids Phospholipids
Phase II	Glucorinidation (most common) Glutathione Conjugation Sulfation Acetylation Methylation Conjugation with Amino Acids	N-acetylcysteine (NAC) Glycine Taurine Glutamine Cysteine Methionine

Antioxidants Used Between Phase I and Phase II

Antioxidants	Found in
Vitamin A	Liver, Mackerel, Salmon, Carrots, Tuna, Butternut Squash, Sweet Potato, Spinach, Broccoli, Red Peppers, Mango, Cantaloupe[202]
Vitamin C	Citrus fruit, Peppers, Strawberries, Blackcurrants, Broccoli, Brussels sprouts, Potatoes, Guava, Thyme, Parsley, Kiwis, Lychees, Persimmons, Papayas

Antioxidants	Found in
Vitamin E	Nuts & Seeds, Salmon, Avocado, Trout, Peppers, Brazil Nuts, Mango, Turnip greens, Kiwis
Selenium	Brazil nuts, Tuna, Oysters, Clams, Halibut, Shrimp, Salmon, Crab, Beef, Pork, Turkey, Chicken, Eggs, Cheese, Mushrooms, Seeds, Spinach, Lentils, Yogurt
Copper	Liver, Oysters, Spirulina, Shiitake Mushrooms, Nuts & Seeds, Lobster
Zinc	Beef, Lamb, Pork, Oysters, Crab, Mussels, Shrimp, Legumes, Seeds, Dairy, Eggs, Whole Grains
Manganese	Mussels, Wheat Germ, Tofu, Sweet Potatoes, Pine Nuts, Brown Rice, Lima Beans, Chickpeas, Spinach, Pineapple
Coenzyme Q10	Liver, Kidney, Sardines, Salmon, Trout, Mackerel, Chicken, Beef, Pork, Spinach, Broccoli, Cauliflower, Fruits, Soybeans, Lentils, Pistachio, Sesame Seeds, Whole Grains
Thiols	Garlic, Onions, Cruciferous vegetables
Bioflavonoids	Berries, Red Cabbage, Onions, Kale, Parsley, Tea, Dark Chocolate, Red Peppers, Citrus Fruit, Mango, Papaya, Garlic, Spinach
Silymarin	Milk Thistle, Artichokes, Grapes, Beet Greens, Berries

Genetics

Phase I reactions are mainly catalyzed by what's called the Cytochrome P450 (CYP) system, which—in plain English—are proteins that detox. Anyone who has gotten into the world of genetics testing has probably seen codes like CYP1B1, CYP2A6, CYP2B6, CYP2C8, CYP2C9, CYP2C19, CYP2D6, CYP2E1, CYP3A4/5/7 (these abbreviations represent different proteins in the CYP450 system). Many of these genetic tests are meant to look where you have SNPs (single nucleotide polymorphisms) in these proteins. A SNP is a common genetic variation and we all have them. What is meant to be gathered from this information is impaired detox. A SNP in the CYP450 system equals inability to detox. I'm not very fond of these tests, because patients order them on their own and then get presented with massive amounts of information, and usually show up at our appointments panicking that they cannot detox. As someone who believes that the most important part of health is mental, emotional, and spiritual health, I think these tests do more harm than good. The information overload often causes cortisol to increase, causing sugar to increase, causing insulin to go up. And as you now know, the two hormones we don't want too much of are cortisol and insulin. So, very simply, my attitude is this: *who cares what your detox genetics look like, do you have elevated toxic burden?*

I would prefer to test you for toxins and if they are elevated, I will simply help you detox, regardless of your prior disposition—and if your levels of toxins are not elevated, I am not going to recommend you detox, regardless of your genetics. If you have less effective detox genetics, could it make you more susceptible for toxins to build up in your body? Sure, but at the end of the day what matters most is reducing your total toxic burden. You will hear different opinions from different practitioners about this, and some may encourage you to get your genetics tested and treat your SNPs with supplements. While people find success in both approaches, my medical practice has had more success when focusing on toxic burden and not genetics.

The most famous SNP seems to be in the gene which codes for the MTHFR enzyme. This enzyme is responsible for the process of methylation in every cell of your body. Methylation is responsible for Phase II detox, cellular repair, production and repair of DNA and mRNA, neurotransmitter production, and healthy immune system function (i.e., formation and maturation of red blood cells, white blood cells and platelet production), so it's a very big deal. When I first learned about it, I thought it was the answer to everything! That's the way it can feel, when you see all its functions. But I've never seen anyone's symptoms go away from just supporting methylation (usually done through supplementing methylated B vitamins). We have so many other reactions happening in our body that when I just focus on one, this has turned out to have a lower yield of accuracy. One of my favorite stories is: I had a patient call me, when I used to be my own receptionist when I was just starting, and he said, "Hey, do you deal with that MT, MTH, MTFHR... the motherfucker gene?" I laughed so hard. When you dive deep, the Internet can really earn the same label, but in my view, there are bigger stones to turn.

Phase I and II Continued

The ongoing process of Phase I and II detox is basically changing the chemical makeup of compounds. This is what our bodies do all over the place: it is basically our metabolic activity. Now let's look at what is happening during the Phase I and II reactions:

Phase I	Reaction	Examples
Oxidation	Addition of oxygen and or removal of hydrogen	R-H $\Rightarrow$ R-OH (R means "Radical Group" meaning any group in which a carbon or hydrogen atom is attached to the rest of the molecule)[203]
Reduction	Addition of hydrogen and or removal of oxygen	R-OH $\Rightarrow$ R-H
Hydrolysis	A reaction with water (H2O) where a toxic compound is broken into two: one compound gets a hydrogen group and the other gets hydroxide (-OH)	R-COO-R' + H2O $\Rightarrow$ R-COOH + R'-OH

This brings back the good ole' days of organic and biochemistry, my legit favorite subjects during pre-med classes. Compounds are labeled as organic or inorganic, where most organic compounds contain carbon and hydrogen, but they may also include any number of other elements, including nitrogen, oxygen, halogens, phosphorus, silicon, sulfur. Examples of organic compounds are: our DNA, table sugar, methane gas, and ethanol. Inorganic compounds are compounds like salts, metals, single element substances, and anything that doesn't contain carbon. Examples of inorganic compounds are table salt, carbon dioxide, diamonds, and silver. Our body can alter compounds by adding or removing these elements like we see above, to make the compounds do different things:

Phase II		
Glucorinidation (most common)	The transfer of glucuronic acid to a substrate by an enzyme called UDP-glucuronosyltransferase	R-C-OH $\Rightarrow$ R-C-O-glucoronyl
Glutathione Conjugation	Enzymes called Glutathione S Transferases add glutathione to toxins to make them water soluble	R + GSH $\Rightarrow$ R-GSH
Sulfation	The addition of sulfur trioxide (SO3)	R + SO3 $\Rightarrow$ R-SO3
Acetylation	The addition of an acetyl group (CH3CO)	R + CH3CO $\Rightarrow$ R-CH3CO
Methylation	The addition of a methyl group (CH3)	R + CH3 $\Rightarrow$ R-CH3
Conjugation with Amino Acids	Combining amino acids with toxic compounds to make them less harmful	The most common amino acids that toxins conjugate with are aspartate and glutamate

Keeping things simple, Phase I and II of detox mostly happens in the liver's hepatocytes, where it is taking compounds which could be harmful and eliminating them, easy right? [FYI: A small amount of Phase I and Phase II happens outside of the liver specifically in your adipose (fat), gut, kidneys, lungs, and skin.]

So back to that lead. Your skin protected you when you touched the lead-painted wall, yet the lead entered through your gut from your drinking water, but was blocked by your liver, and made water soluble. So, in a safe way, the detoxified lead can now enter the bloodstream and flow to the kidneys, or they can pass with bile into the gut for excretion. The kidneys are your filters, they let water-soluble substances pass through and create your urine, which is then how you pee out the toxins. Since the lead is now water soluble, it can leave through your sweat as well. If instead the neutralized toxins attach to bile and get pushed inside of your intestine (which is technically outside of your body), the toxin has now left your body and you can send it all the way out when you poop. For this reason, some call the gut "phase III of detox." Yet as toxins are flowing through your gut, they can be reabsorbed. Why? It is normal for bile acids to be reabsorbed. Or, what if you have leaky gut? If your gut barrier is lost then those toxins can just flow right back in, and pass through the liver again.

Lymphatics

What about bacteria, viruses, cancerous cells, and other pathogens? There are specific cells called Kuppfer cells in your liver. They are a special type of macrophage and part of your innate immunity, engulfing pathogens and giving them the boot through a healthy immune response. Did you know that the lymphatic system circulates about twice as much fluid as your cardiovascular system? Your immune system is everywhere, so it is not just in your liver that macrophages are protecting you; it's happening all around your body. You also have over 600 lymph nodes, which are sites where pathogens can be trapped and neutralized by the innate and adaptive immune systems. Pathogens that have been wiped out by the immune system then pass into the blood for excretion.

Lungs

We often think about lungs in terms of our breath, but not so much in terms of their role as a detox organ. The lungs are where oxygen and carbon dioxide leave and enter, and they are also one of our most vital detox organs. Let's say that lead from airplane exhaust tries to enter through your respiratory system. The lungs produce mucus, which traps particles trying to get in. Your airways are lined with tiny hairs called cilia. Cilia move back and forth, sweeping mucus out of your lungs and into your throat. When you cough up a bunch of phlegm, you are clearing toxins and pathogens from your body.

At the end of your airways are your alveoli. We have about 480 million alveoli, and this is where gas exchange happens. Alveoli expand to let oxygen in your blood and contract when you breathe out carbon dioxide. The alveoli are another barrier and should not let toxins and pathogens across. But what if your alveoli are inflamed or leaky (i.e., from smoking cigarettes)? Just as within the gut, the barrier is lost, so can be the respiratory system's shield. Toxins or pathogens that were not excreted by the skin, liver, kidneys, or gut can be pushed out through the alveoli and into the mucus to be coughed out.

Smoking is not as cool as some once thought it was, but there are still people doing it. What does seem to be more cool right now is vaping, which is advertised as a "safer" alternative to cigarettes; I respectfully disagree and think vaping may actually be even worse for you. There are many books and studies supporting how damaging smoking is to human health. In the context of detox, smoking destroys the alveoli. And FYI, alveoli don't grow back, so when you destroy them, you have permanently destroyed part of your lungs. If someone smokes long enough, destroying more and more alveoli, the disease emphysema develops. There are also more than 7,000 chemicals in tobacco smoke, where at least 250 are known to be harmful,[204] and nearly 2,000 chemicals found in vaping aerosols.[205] Remember the first step in detox is always to stop your toxic exposure.

Our Toxic World

Wow! There we have it, detoxification simplified. Our bodies are amazing, aren't they? So how do people get so "toxic?" Unfortunately, our food industry, pharmaceutical industry, transportation industry, not to mention pathogens (e.g., viruses, bacteria, and mold); and just in general, technological advances (the things we use for home and building construction, smart phones, WIFI, etc.) have taken our bodies amazing abilities for granted. In the generation of more and more profits and power, corporations and governments have focused on making things bigger, stronger, faster, and better, without really ever paying attention to how it affects human beings.

Cancer prevalence in the United States was 3.6 million people in 1975, in 2040 the number is expected to be 26.1 million.[206]

In 1958 1.6 million people in the United States were diagnosed with Diabetes, in 2015 23.4 million were diagnosed with Diabetes.[207]

The worldwide obesity rate has nearly tripled since 1975, 650 million adults worldwide were obese.[208]

The rate of autism was 2 to 4 out of every 10,000 children in the 1960s,[209] yet in 2021 the rate was 1 out of every 44 children…[210]

There are no causation studies that report our environment as the sole cause, but there is a strong correlation with what we have done to our food, bodies, and minds with respect to the rise of chronic disease. Let's look at reasons someone may become toxic.

Too Much Exposure

Our bodies can all get rid of a certain amount of toxins a day. If my body could get rid of 100 toxins per day, and in an average day I am only exposed to 75 toxins, my detox mechanisms should be able to keep up. But let's say someone starts binge drinking on the weekends, eating fast food and sushi 3 times per week, stays in denial about trauma they have experienced in the past, moves into a moldy apartment, sleeps with their phone by the bed, and drinks tap water full of lead, and now their body is exposed to 10,000 toxins per day. In theory, 9,900 will get stored. Their skin, gut, liver, kidneys, lungs, and lymphatic system will try to protect them, but the organs and systems become overwhelmed, so that fat-soluble toxins will find places to hang out in the body's tissues.

And let's say they're 20 years old and healthy when this started, with no symptoms to report. Over the years, when they develop gut issues and headaches, they go to their doctor, who does routine testing and tells them everything is fine and gives them medications to feel better. But those meds just increased the toxic load and put a Band-Aid on symptoms without the person ever questioning it. Then they hit their mid-40s and their joints are super stiff, so they go back to their doctor and this time everything is not fine; they diagnose them with

Rheumatoid Arthritis and prescribe an immunosuppressive drug (even more toxic). The drug helps at first and then stops working, so now the doctor recommends a second drug, but the patient has had enough, turns to Dr. Google, and boom! They find Functional Medicine!

Their Functional Medicine doctor identifies the root causes (i.e., exotoxins like mercury from the sushi and lead from the water, fats and sugar from their diet, mold mycotoxins from their apartment, and EMF exposure—not to mention endotoxins from their gut and the trauma they've never dealt with). Eureka! They finally have an explanation for the pain in their joints: their toxic burden was overwhelmed, their bucket overflowed.

In my experience as Functional Medicine doctor, the symptoms from an elevated toxic burden can be *anything*. As we saw, they can travel all over the body, so I can take 100 patients with elevated lead and they all have different symptoms, or none at all yet. The same goes for any toxic burden; it creates inflammation all over the body, and symptoms can be different for everyone and can change over time. What are some other reasons a person can become toxic? Here are a few common risks for being more susceptible to toxins:

	Causes
Leaky Skin	Excess sun exposure, Standard American Diet, dehydration, cigarettes and alcohol, and environmental toxins
Leaky Gut	Stress, dysbiosis, environmental toxins, low stomach acid, Standard American Diet, SIBO, drugs and alcohol
Suppressed Immune Response	Stress, Standard American Diet, lack of sleep, poor gut health, lack of nutrition, drugs and alcohol
Leaky Lungs	Cigarette smoking, vaping, chronic marijuana use, chronic lung infections

	Causes
Inflamed Liver	Excess toxic burden, blocked bile flow, Standard American Diet, medications, drugs and alcohol
Clogged Kidneys	High blood sugar, high blood pressure, heavy toxic exposure, drugs and alcohol
Poor Nutrition or Digestion	There are so many vitamins and minerals used in detox (see above); if you are not getting enough of them from your diet or you're not digesting, you will not absorb them
Genetics	SNPs in enzymes and proteins which are responsible for detox

The overarching theme here? Your ability to detox lies in your ability to live a healthy lifestyle in a toxic world—but fortunately, you can make your corner of that world less toxic by making good decisions. Most people inhibit their detox, rather support it—but you can choose differently, because of your new awareness of the facts. Once the toxins are stored in the body, how do they contribute to disease? Here are some ways:

- Damage DNA
- Modify Gene Expression
- Poison enzymes
- Damage organs
- Impair detox ability
- Break cell membranes
- Create hormone damage

Yet it doesn't have to get to this point—that is what this book is for. Now that you have an idea of how your body is built to protect you, let's look at some of the most common toxin issues, which your body may be dealing with even while you're unaware of them: heavy metals, mold mycotoxins, and household toxins. By becoming conscious of what you didn't know, you begin to heal and strengthen your detox ability. So let's keep going!

CHAPTER 7

Heavy Metals

Before we dig in to the world of heavy metals, here's the most important fact to know: not all heavy metals are problematic. Some heavy metals are essential nutrients, like iron, cobalt, and zinc, but these are not our topic here. What we are going to focus on is the environmental toxic metals, which even at low levels can contribute to disease. Some common examples that can be problematic even at low levels are lead and mercury. And most metals, whether they are essential or not, can become toxic at high levels, such as chromium and vanadium. First, we are going to talk about the individual metals, how you get them, what they can do to your body, how you test for them, and how you can get them out. Then we'll look at a couple of my patient case studies. Remember, toxins like metals can cause disease because they can:

- Damage DNA
- Modify gene expression
- Poison enzymes
- Damage organs
- Impair detox ability
- Break cell membranes
- Damage hormones

The specific effects of a toxin on a cell are as follows:

The toxin acts on cells and mitochondria by inducing oxidative stress (inflammation) and generating reactive oxygen species (ROS), activating apoptosis (cell death), inhibiting the electron transport chain (energy production), reducing ATP synthesis (energy), altering membrane permeability, and damaging DNA and proteins.

This process holds true for heavy metals. What's amazing is that traditional medicine agrees with us. According to an article in *Molecular, Clinical and Environmental Toxicology*:

> Their toxicity depends on several factors including the dose, route of exposure, and chemical species, as well as the age, gender, genetics, and nutritional status of exposed individuals. Because of their high degree of toxicity, arsenic, cadmium, chromium, lead, and mercury rank among the priority metals that are of public health significance. These metallic elements are considered systemic toxicants that are known to induce multiple organ damage, even at lower levels of exposure. They are also classified as human carcinogens (known or probable) according to the U.S. Environmental Protection Agency, and the International Agency for Research on Cancer.[211]

So why doesn't your regular doctor test you? I don't know the answer for sure. I think it has to do with the pharmaceutical industry, but we'll discuss this soon. Let's start with lead, the most common toxic heavy metal I see in my practice.

Lead

According to the United States Environmental Protection Agency (EPA):

> Lead is a naturally occurring element found in small amounts in the earth's crust. Lead can be found in all

parts of our environment—the air, the soil, the water, and even inside our homes. Much of our exposure comes from human activities including the use of fossil fuels including past use of leaded gasoline, some types of industrial facilities and past use of lead-based paint in homes. Lead and its compounds have been used in a wide variety of products found in and around our homes, including paint, ceramics, pipes and plumbing materials, solders, gasoline, batteries, ammunition and cosmetics. Lead may enter the environment from these past and current uses. Lead can also be emitted into the environment from industrial sources and contaminated sites, such as former lead smelters. While natural levels of lead in soil range between 50 and 400 parts per million, mining, smelting and refining activities have resulted in substantial increases in lead levels in the environment, especially near mining and smelting sites.

When lead is released to the air from industrial sources or spark-ignition engine aircraft, it may travel long distances before settling to the ground, where it usually sticks to soil particles. Lead may move from soil into ground water depending on the type of lead compound and the characteristics of the soil.[212]

So it's literally everywhere! No wonder I find levels built up in the majority of people I test. The traditional medicine side mainly identifies children and pregnant women as at risk, with lead toxicity causing things like behavior and learning problems, lower IQ, slow growth, miscarriage, pre-term delivery, and organ damage to the unborn infant. In my experience, everyone is at risk for secondary effects to lead. It is linked to cardiovascular effects like increased blood pressure (according to the CDC, nearly *half* of adults in the United States, about 116 million people, have hypertension;[213] also see the case study of Jerry's High Blood Pressure on page 132), and decreased kidney function (impaired detox as we just learned), along with reproductive problems (hormone imbalances as discussed in Chapters 1 through 6).

Mercury

The second most common toxic metal I find built up in people is mercury. According to the EPA, "Mercury is a naturally occurring chemical element found in rock in the earth's crust, including within deposits of coal."[214] It exists in several forms: elemental mercury, inorganic mercury compounds, and methylmercury.

Elemental mercury is a shiny, silver-white metal, historically referred to as quicksilver, and is liquid at room temperature. It is used in older thermometers, fluorescent lightbulbs, and some electrical switches.[215]

Inorganic mercury occurs abundantly in the environment and can combine with other elements to form inorganic mercury salts. These salts can be transported in water and occur in soil, and it can get to these places through air as a byproduct of mining. Mercury salts are used in skin-lightening creams, photography, disinfectants (think about the use of these since the pandemic started), wood preservatives, fungicides, and in the coloring of paints and tattoo dyes (don't worry if you see my arms; my artist used only organic dyes). Emissions of both elemental and inorganic mercury can occur from coal-fired power plants, waste burning, and from factories that use mercury.

Methylmercury occurs due to the constant reshuffling of mercury in the environment. Mercury salts get attached to airborne particles. Rain and snow deposit these on the ground, and then it returns to the atmosphere as a gas. The mercury then undergoes biochemical transformations, very similar to what phase I and phase II of detox looked like, making it organic and highly toxic. Nearly ALL methylmercury exposures in the United States occur through eating fish and shellfish that contain higher levels of methylmercury. Once in the air, mercury eventually settles into bodies of water like oceans, lakes and streams, or onto land, where it can be washed by runoff into larger bodies of water. Microorganisms in waterbodies can change it into methylmercury, where it builds up in fish and shellfish. The highest active levels of Mercury I have seen in patients is those eating sushi three or more times per week. I love sushi myself—I even got to have fresh-off-the-boat sushi for breakfast at Tsukiji Market in Tokyo, Japan—I just try to limit it. Daily ingestion of fish can result in the assimilation of 1 to 10 micrograms of mercury per day.

So, as you can see, methylmercury is another toxic metal that is virtually everywhere! And again, not shocking that I find elevations in so many people.

Two places the EPA does not mention where mercury can be found are dental amalgams (mercury fillings) and some vaccines in the form of thimerosal. On the FDA website, they are very clear to point out that they've tried to remove it from most vaccines or offer an option that does not have it, but they don't believe it's an issue for anyone. The most common vaccine which has thimerosal is the influenza vaccine, as well as tetanus and diphtheria toxoids. According to the FDA, "there is a robust body of peer-reviewed, scientific studies conducted in the United States and countries around the world that support the safety of thimerosal-containing vaccines. The scientific evidence collected over the past 15 years does not show any evidence of harm, including serious neurodevelopmental disorders, from use of thimerosal in vaccines."[216] Have I worked with many families who say 100% their child was never the same after some vaccinations? Yes, many. Regular people who have had vaccines or mercury fillings say yes, they've had detrimental health effects, governmental agencies say no, mercury fillings and vaccines do not have negative side effects, it is a very sensitive subject, I am not saying yes or no, I am just providing information and my experience of working with patients with chronic disease. If you are interested in working with a mercury-safe dentist who has experience with amalgam removal, find one at the International Academy of Oral Medicine and Toxicology: www.iaomt.org.

Cesium and Thallium

I think these two will blow your mind. For years, I had been seeing higher and higher elevation in cesium and thallium, and then one specific patient helped me put it together. Let's learn about the metals first.

The most common uses for cesium compounds are as a drilling fluid, to make special optical glass, and as a catalyst promoter, in vacuum tubes and in radiation monitoring equipment. One of its most important uses is in the "cesium clock" (atomic clock). These clocks are a vital part of the internet and mobile phone networks, as well as Global Positioning System (GPS) satellites.

Thallium is considered one of the most toxic metals there is. It's estimated that approximately 500 tons of the thallium are released into environment every year, mostly from combustion of coal, where the particles get into the air and settle in our soil.[217] It also comes from the refinery of petroleum and drilling for oil. Wheat and corn can accumulate 55mg/kg of thallium. Why are they showing up in so many of my patients? It happens through their wheat, corn, vegetable and fruit consumption, because cesium and thallium get into our soil and our crops absorb them.

I had a family who brought in their 8-year-old child to work up underlying causes of obsessive-compulsive behaviors. If there are no gut symptoms and there are neurologic or behavioral issues, I will typically start with toxins. So we tested his heavy metal levels and they all came back within normal limits, but the cesium and thallium were extremely elevated. What stuck out to me the most at the initial visit is this child's diet. He had never eaten gluten, dairy, soy, corn, or eggs, and his diet was extremely healthy based on most people's criteria. He ate a lot of vegetables and fruit, a lot! So when we got his results back, I was shocked and I did a consult with a doctor at the lab I ordered testing from. They explained what they have been seeing: patients with the highest levels of vegetable and fruit intake had the highest cesium and thallium levels. Mind blown. In Central California, oil companies in 2013 produced 150 million barrels of oil—and nearly 2 billion barrels of wastewater. Farms, including "organic" farms experiencing droughts, use this wastewater to irrigate their crops. According to the article, researchers don't know the long-term toxicity of up to 80 percent of the hundreds of materials used in oilfield production. [218] Well, I think I am seeing it in my practice. This water has cesium and thallium in it. These toxins are invading our crops from every direction and, in turn, our bodies.

Arsenic

I don't see a lot of elevated arsenic levels. I think it's due to the limits of testing, because it is another heavy metal that is extremely prevalent. According to the EPA, arsenic is a naturally occurring element widely distributed in the earth's crust. In the environment, arsenic is combined with oxygen, chlorine, and sulfur to form inorganic arsenic compounds. Arsenic in animals and plants combines with carbon and hydrogen to form organic arsenic compounds. Inorganic arsenic compounds are mainly used to preserve wood (think pressure-treated lumber). Organic arsenic compounds are used as pesticides, primarily on cotton fields and orchards. Arsenic is also found in cigarettes.[219] The WHO says the greatest threat to public health from arsenic originates from contaminated groundwater—namely, drinking it and consuming crops irrigated with water that has arsenic— but fish, shellfish, meat, poultry, dairy products and cereals can also be dietary sources of arsenic.[220]

Both organizations go on to say almost nothing is known regarding health effects of organic arsenic compounds in humans. They do say there is some evidence that long-term exposure to arsenic in children may result in lower IQ scores. There is also some evidence that exposure to arsenic in the womb and early childhood may increase mortality in young adults. There is further evidence that inhaled or ingested arsenic can injure pregnant women or their unborn babies, although the studies are not conclusive. From my standpoint, a toxin is a toxin, and if it is filling your bucket, I would want to limit it or get rid of it.

Other Metals

The rest of the metals that I find from time to time in patients are: barium, bismuth, and gadolinium. Barium and gadolinium usually come from people who have done imaging studies (i.e., procedures like a barium swallow or upper GI series) and gadolinium from MRIs with contrast. So your traditional doctor is going to argue that they're safe. It's up to you to educate yourself.

Barium

Frozen and fast foods (such as burgers, fries, and hot dogs), Brazil nuts and peanuts/peanut butter are very high in barium, so it can be high if you test after eating these foods. It can also enter the air during coal and oil combustion. Barium compounds are used by the oil and gas industries to make drilling mud, which makes drilling easier. Barium compounds are also used to make paint, bricks, tiles, glass, and rubber. Soluble barium compounds are highly toxic and may be used as insecticides. So this is another one that is just about everywhere. Is it an issue? From the traditional standpoint, no, unless you have really high levels. From a Functional standpoint, it's a toxin that can contribute to your toxic load.

Gadolinium

Besides its use in MRIs, gadolinium is often used in alloys like chromium and iron, the phosphors of color TV, and in making magnets and electronic components (such as recording heads for video recorders), computer memory, and in the manufacture of compact disks, though I'm not sure these are made anymore. Gadolinium has no known biological role in humans. Toxicity is rarely associated with gadolinium due to poor gut absorption. I only find high levels in those people who have had an MRI, but I have never seen it be an issue on its own.

Bismuth

Most people would be familiar with bismuth from the over-the-counter (OTC) product "Pepto-Bismol." Bismuth has therapeutic uses with antimicrobial, anti-secretory and anti-inflammatory properties, and it was used to treat syphilis.

Bismuth is also a byproduct of lead and copper ore refining. The existence of health problems due to environmental pollution by bismuth is not documented. At low levels, no toxic effects are documented for bismuth. Due to my experience of seeing the magic happen with patients who get the func out, I would be careful if you have become reliant on OTC products containing bismuth. By following the steps in *Unfunc Your Gut*, I think people can get off of it.

More Metals

The other metals that are included when patients do a toxic metal urine profile with me are: aluminum, antimony, beryllium, cadmium, nickel, palladium, platinum, tellurium, thorium, tin, tungsten, and uranium. Since I rarely find these, I don't think they are high yield enough to discuss. If you have suffered toxicity as a result of any of these metals, know that there is help and it is possible to get the func out.

Testing

If you're worried that you have an issue with heavy metals, what can you do? I always start with testing, because I don't think people should play a guessing game with their life. In my experience the more convinced someone is that they have something, the less likely they are to test positive for that thing. Reading the beginning of this chapter, I think you can see that we are all at risk for having a heavy metal issue. So how can you find out?

Start by going back and looking at any traditional lab testing you've had done. For example, looking at a CBC (complete blood count). A common finding I see is a low white blood cell count. When I see this, I am definitely going to test to rule out toxins as an underlying issue. Why would toxins cause a low white blood cell count? As we have mentioned many times, toxins cause cell death and can specifically target your immune cells. White blood cells are one of the main cells of your immune response.

Another common test that your doctor may have ordered is a CMP (comprehensive metabolic profile), which includes liver function tests (LFT), or patients may have ordered LFTs on their own. The markers to pay attention too are ALT, AST, alkaline phosphatase, albumin, total protein, and bilirubin to assess liver inflammation and function. If these markers are imbalanced, your doctor probably then tested you for the different types of hepatitis; and if those came back negative, they probably told you not to worry. If these markers are imbalanced, I would take it one step further and test for your toxins. Remember, your liver is your main detox organ, so if it is overworked due to toxicity, it may show up inflamed on lab testing.

There are also other serum markers, including GGT, LD, PT, PTT, and INR, that you may have had checked in the past. GGT is an enzyme found primarily in liver. It is part of the glutathione pathway, and it is the most sensitive marker of liver disease; and in the Functional Medicine world, it's considered a possible marker for oxidative stress when it is elevated. It goes up due to things like alcohol, meds, high blood sugar, high thyroid, and toxins. When it's elevated, it could mean more glutathione is being used.

Glutathione is your body's master antioxidant—it gets used up when your body is trying to get rid of toxins.

Bilirubin could be elevated in someone with impaired bile flow.

Albumin and **Total Protein** would be low in chronic liver damage.

PT, PTT, and INR will rise in people with severe liver disease, because the liver is not making sufficient clotting factors.

Going back and looking at some of the lab tests you've had done can be helpful. I will frequently order these tests for patients, but I do not find them that helpful. **That is because all of your traditional lab testing may come back normal, even if you still have elevated levels of toxins.**

There are labs for measuring oxidative stress. We can check levels of glutathione, lipid peroxides, glutathione peroxidase, 8-hydroxy-deoxyguanosine (8-OH-DG in the urine) and superoxide dismutase. These kinds of tests will give you a better picture of whether or not your body is inflamed. If these markers come back imbalanced, it still leaves us with the question, *why are they imbalanced?* Which is why I like to jump straight to the point and measure toxin levels, because toxins can be present even when you are not showing up with inflammation.

We can also test your gut to learn about how you're detoxing through a comprehensive stool analysis. There is a marker in a comprehensive stool analysis called β-Glucuronidase, and it is relevant to detox because it is a marker that could mean you're reabsorbing toxins. Glucuronidation is phase II reaction that can send toxins out into your gut for excretion. If β-Glucuronidase is present, it can react with the toxin, basically counteracting what your liver did, making the toxin active again and causing you to reabsorb it. We can lower levels of β-Glucuronidase by unfunc'ing your gut.

Heavy Metal Testing

Now this is one area where I was trained very differently as a traditional doctor versus a Functional Medicine doctor. In traditional medicine we are taught to use blood testing to evaluate a patient suspected of having heavy metal poisoning. This a fantastic test if you're worried about acute exposure. You can measure lead and mercury through blood testing and if there was significant exposure in the prior few months it will come back high.[221] Lead in the blood has a very short half-life, about 35 days, so the exposure must be recent to catch it in the blood. Urine testing is also very good at catching recent exposure, for example it is the best way to assess acute arsenic exposure.

One type of testing used frequently in the alternative medicine world is hair testing. When I first started my career I would order it, but quickly found it to be virtually useless. Data is insufficient to predict health effects from the concentration of the substance in hair. It can be affected by substances used for hair treatment. There are not enough validity, reliability, and reference range tests to support hair testing.[222] I have never used it, but it's possible to use stool testing for mercury, cadmium, lead, antimony and uranium exposure, as a marker of acute exposure. But at the end of the day, if you're worried about acute exposure, you should be going to the emergency room, not reaching out to my office. What I can help you with is your total toxic body burden (i.e., the lifetime accumulation of a little bit of lead, mercury, arsenic, etc.). Your total toxic load could be presenting as Hashimoto's, Lupus, high blood pressure, brain fog or any other kind of chronic issues. Maybe you feel terrible but your doctor tells you all your tests are normal and to try an anti-depressant. Sound familiar?

Pre- and Post-Chelation Testing

Pre- and post-chelation testing is my preferred choice for diagnosing heavy metal toxic burden. If you asked me, "What is the number one test you would order for someone as a preventative medicine test?"—it would be this. Yes, even though I wrote my first book about gut health, and that is usually why people come to me, if I didn't know anything about someone's history, I would start with heavy metals. Why? Because as you have been learning they are very prevalent: in much of the air we breathe, the food we eat, and many of the things we touch. And as you also learned, they can be highly damaging to our body. Honestly, this a tough stance to take as a Medical Doctor, because the traditional medical community is not behind this.

Before I explain why, let's take a look: what is pre- and post-chelation testing? It is the analysis of toxic metal levels in urine after administering a metal detoxification agent as an objective way to evaluate the accumulation of toxic metals. Acute metal poisoning (what traditional doctors test for) is rare. However, what we've been talking about is toxic burden, a chronic, low-level exposure to toxic metals that can result in significant retention in the body, and that can be associated with a vast array of adverse health effects and chronic disease. For an individual, toxicity occurs when more toxins accumulate than your body can eliminate. To evaluate this net retention, we compare the levels of metals in urine before and after the administration of a pharmaceutical metal detoxification agent such as EDTA, DMSA or DMPS.[1] These medications act by sequestering "hidden" metals from deep tissue stores and mobilizing the metals to the kidneys for excretion in the urine.

It is a two-part test. The initial test is just a random first morning urine that measures recent or ongoing exposure. Then you take a dose of chelating agent prescribed by your doctor. It is based on weight (I typically use DMSA at 30mg/kg).[223] The chelating agent is pulling out what is stored in your body and you are collecting urine for 6 hours after. My preferred lab for this test is called Doctor's Data and you're given a big orange jug

---

1   Ethylenediaminetetraacetic acid, dimercaptosuccinic acid, or dimercap-
     to-propane sulfonate.

to collect urine samples over a 6-hour period. A day of collecting the sample would look like this:

Step 1. The pre-test. Wake up and pee in a cup. This should be your first urination of the morning; let's say this is at 6 a.m. Follow the instructions in your lab kit and then send your sample via FedEx (or similar) to the lab. This is your pre-test.

Step 2. Take your DMSA, let's say at 6:15 a.m. Wait until you have to pee; let's say next time is 8 a.m. Collect this urine in a cup provided and transfer it to the big orange jug, which you keep in the fridge. This is when you set your 6-hour timer, and every time you pee after that you collect it and transfer it to the jug. After you're done, at 2 p.m. in this example, you shake up your jug and transfer a specimen into a vial and send it to the lab. This is your post-test.

Your Functional Medicine doctor will interpret the results for you. Seems easy enough, right? And after all you have learned about toxins and how they affect your body, wouldn't you want to know what your toxic burden is? Why your regular doctor will not support this, I don't know, but here are two articles I found that discuss it:

> In summary, current evidence does not support the use of DMPS, DMSA, or other chelation challenge tests for the diagnosis of metal toxicity. Since there are no established reference ranges for provoked urine samples in healthy subjects, no reliable evidence to support a diagnostic value for the tests, and potential harm, these tests should not be utilized.[224]

And another one:

As academic toxicologists, we are increasingly con-
sulted by patients anxious about their recent diagnosis
of heavy metal poisoning based on the results of an
overpriced post chelation testing. Even safer alternatives,
such as DMSA or DMPS, may increase the elimination
of certain essential elements, and side effects include
abdominal distress, transient rash, elevated circulating
liver transaminases, and neutropenia. This may not
be significant when used for a single provocation test,
but the problem may become important for patients
enrolled in successive chelation cures to rid their body
of a toxic burden.[225]

They did mention a little later in the article:

Chelating agents are great drugs when used wisely, and
excellent reviews are available on the topic.[226]

From the alternative medicine side, Dr. Walter Crinnion published a study which argued that measuring urine heavy metals
is an accepted method for assessing the presence of these toxins
in an individual.[227]

When I first learned about pre and post heavy metal testing,
coming at it from a traditional side, I was concerned and did
not use this testing. No one had ever talked to me about it as an
option, so it was unknown. But I spent more time learning about
Environmental Medicine and became convinced it sounded like
a reasonable strategy.

In response to the articles that I referenced, there are a
couple things I want to comment on, the first being what they
called "the high cost." This almost made me fall out of my chair
laughing. A urine heavy metal test can range around $100 and
the chelating agent price varies by pharmacy and quantity

ordered; a 6-month chelation plan, including supplements, can be done for under $1,000. Did anyone else reading this have any experience with traditional medicine? Does anything cost $100 to $1,000? The costs are mind-blowing in the traditional medicine world, insofar as what they charge for basic lab tests let alone doctor visits, hospital stays, medications etc.

While spending $1,000 up front can be overwhelming, consider it in the grand scheme of things as $1000 to help prevent a lifetime of diseases. Here's just one example: a new Alzheimer's drug was controversially approved by the FDA. In 2020, the original asking price for one year of treatment was over $50,000. Due to backlash in 2021, they lowered the price to $28,200.[228] The financial burden of chronic disease is staggering. In 2016, the total costs in the U.S. for direct health care treatment of chronic health conditions totaled $1.1 trillion.[229] And these reports were complaining about the cost of a urine heavy metal test or a chelating agent? Get the func out!

In regard to there not being established reference ranges, I don't totally disagree. But should we have any toxic heavy metals in our body at all? Our bodies were not meant to accumulate toxins. One could argue that anything above zero is outside of reference range. Doctors Data, the lab that I use, says; "Results are creatinine corrected to account for urine dilution variations. Reference intervals are based upon NHANES (cdc.gov/nhanes) data if available, and are representative of a large population cohort under non-provoked conditions. Chelation (provocation) agents can increase urinary excretion of metals/elements." For example the reference interval for lead <1.2 and mercury <1.3.

Yes, I agree that every medication has side effects, yet the main problem with DMSA is that it also leaches vitamins and minerals out of your body. So, taking it every day or at high doses could be extremely dangerous, just like with anything. I have taken thousands of people through chelation therapy and never did anyone have anything beyond mild symptoms, such as abdominal pain or fatigue. However, it is definitely not for everyone; I've worked with a number of patients who could not tolerate it at all. We usually know this on test day. If someone cannot tolerate the test day, we will not do chelation therapy.

So what does the whole process look like? Let's look at a remarkable patient I worked with, so you can get a better picture of what chelation entails.

A Case Study in Chelation: Jerry's High Blood Pressure

When Jerry first came in to visit me, he was 62 years old. As always, my first question was: what are your goals or expectations from working with me? Jerry said he was coming in for better health; besides some fatigue and muscle and joint pain, he felt good on a day-to-day basis. He said he felt better at a lower weight and in the past 9 months he had gained 20 pounds, so he wanted to lose some weight. His current diet focus was intermittent fasting; he only ate one big meal per day, he worked a night shift and would snack during work, and he followed a high protein low carb diet.

Jerry was taking 20 different supplements daily based on information he had learned via books and audio (radio and podcasts). When he was younger, he was a body builder and while in the military he'd smoked 1 to 2 packs per day for 14 years. He had a history of GERD, which he had eliminated by cutting out caffeine. He also had a history of high cholesterol and high blood pressure. He was on 3 medications for his blood pressure for over 10 years, including two diuretics and a ACE inhibitor. On this regimen, his blood pressure was very well controlled, ranging in the 110s over 60s. He had lab testing one month earlier after a bout of gout, where they found multiple electrolyte imbalances, but didn't mention why that could be.

Electrolyte imbalances were not surprising to me, being that he was on so many meds, and also could have explained his fatigue and muscle issues.

My first thought was: if we can get him off of his blood pressure meds, everything would get better. Now, what's the easiest way to do this? Lose some weight and detox? I was really focused on toxins as an underlying issue based on his history in the military, the smoking, and his job in the transportation industry. He had not been doing any exercise for the last year, so I thought it was a good idea for him to start again. As a former body builder he agreed. Besides exercise, I recommended an elimination diet (see *Unfunc Your Gut*), pre- and post-chelation heavy metal testing, and focus on healing past traumas with a therapist (also discussed in *Unfunc Your Gut*). Moreover, we stopped almost all of his supplements and just left a multivitamin, fish oil (I bumped his dose of EPA/DHA to 2000mg twice daily), and CoQ10 (I increased his dose to 200mg daily). Most people come to me assuming I'm going to send them to the store with a long shopping list for supplements, but this doesn't happen unless we have testing that indicates a reason to do so. (The overwhelming majority of the time, I'm supporting people in getting people off of supplements. Taking supplements long term is a traditional approach, "a pill for the ill," whereas my focus is to identify root causes and eliminate them. If you have a practitioner who is prescribing you a bunch of supplements without testing and having a plan, I would be careful.) I also advised him to get back with a cardiologist to readjust his blood pressure meds while we were working on underlying issues, to help balance the electrolyte issues.

When Jerry came back 6 weeks later to go over his test results, he was doing about the same, in his opinion. He had not yet started the diet, but he had worked on stress quite a bit by starting to exercise daily and had taken 10 days off of work. He had done his testing correctly, collecting his first morning urine as a pre test, then taking his DMSA one time (Jerry's dose was 2,500mg based on his weight and recommended dosing which is 30mg/kg with a maximum of 2,500mg—DMSA is easiest to find in 500mg capsules, so I usually round up or down to the closest 500mg interval), and collecting his urine for 6 hours after. Here are his results of note:

The Pre-Test

Random Urine	Jerry's Level	Reference Interval
Barium	15	<7
Lead	0.8	<2

Looking at it again, Jerry had one of the best pre-tests I've seen. Usually most people have some cesium and thallium show up here, and occasionally lead or mercury, but he did not. All this indicated to us is that he did not have *acute* toxicity from heavy metals. With this information, a traditional doctor would have been done and told him he did not have a heavy metal issue and to just focus on adjusting his blood pressure meds. But, we have to get the func out! So I looked at his post-chelation test to give us an indication of total toxic body burden. How full was his bucket of heavy metals? My guess was it was that significant:

The Post-Test

6 hour urine post 2,500mg of DMSA	Jerry's Level	Reference Interval
Barium	21	<7
Cadmium	0.7	<0.8
Cesium	9.1	<9
Lead	30	<2
Mercury	0.9	<3
Thallium	0.3	<0.5

For reference, my own lead level was 11 and the highest I've ever seen was over 140 in an airport mechanic. So the argument is, there is no definite reference range and I agree, but I think that is because every one of us is different, and that's where the clinician comes into play. In my experience, the elevation in levels does not correlate with severity of symptoms. I have had patients with severe symptoms at a level of 8 and mild ones at 65. I also can't tell someone with symptoms that they are definitely due to the metals, but it is usually worth it try to find out. How do you that?

Let's look at what happened with Jerry.
Based on Jerry's levels, it appeared he would need a 13-month chelation plan. The only metal that was really worrisome was the lead. (There are different chelating agents available for different metals. DMSA is best for lead; your trusted practitioner can guide you to which is best for you.) I usually use 4, 7, or 13 months as a starting point, depending on what the person's levels are. My own plan was 7 months for a post-chelation lead of 11. Different practitioners have different detox plans; this plan has always served my patients well.

First-Month Antioxidant Loading

- Liposomal glutathione daily (from Readisorb)

- Detox support (Pretty much all the supplement companies make some kind of detox support; they are nutrients that are needed in phase I and II of detox and antioxidants. Some of my favorites are Ultra Clear Renew from Metagenics or, if following a Low FODMAP diet, Detox Support capsules from Pure.)

- Multivitamin daily (Metagenics or Pure)

Second to Thirteenth Month Chelation

- I recommend DMSA once daily for four days (Jerry's dose was 2,500mg, but check with your practitioner).

- During chelation days (while taking DMSA), it's advisable is to increase water intake by 6 glasses of water on days of DMSA.

- He was to take his normal meds or supplements 2 hours apart from DMSA. Otherwise, DMSA would bind onto anything else taken and not be absorbed, essentially making his blood pressure meds ineffective, which would be very dangerous. Reminder: chelation must be done safely under the supervision of a qualified physician!)

- I recommend taking the DMSA in the morning so the body can excrete the toxins throughout the day. If the patient takes it at night, they will either need to wake up every couple hours to pee or those toxins will just sit and get reabsorbed.

- After 4 days, stop the DMSA and take the detox support from month one daily for 10 days.

- Take daily meds regularly.

- After 10 days, start DMSA again for 4 days, rinse and repeat.

- Keep the same regimen going. (This lasted one year for Jerry: 4 days on DMSA to get the toxic metals out and 10 days to restore.)

We discussed the possible side effects of DMSA,[230] which include:

- GI upset (e.g., diarrhea, loose stool, loss of appetite, nausea and vomiting)
- Skin reactions
- Mild neutropenia
- Elevated liver enzymes
- Change in urine odor
- Depletion of nutrients (This is my greatest concern for DMSA treatment and so it's why we load someone before starting therapy and do twice as much replenishing as we do chelation.)

I told Jerry to reach out if he had any issues with treatment and I gave him the option of repeating a post-chelation test after 7 months to check in and see how his chelation is going. Everyone detoxes at a different rate. I have actually seen levels go up after 7 months, which is rare, but the thinking is that the chelation is pulling much more that was stored and not caught on test day out. Jerry liked the plan and was ready to go; he also said he would start to work on his diet as well.

Jerry did not reach out for 13 months. When he did, he asked to repeat a post-chelation test and then schedule a visit. His post chelation lead came back at 4.9 (down from 30). Woohoo! The best part was that he was feeling great, he'd lost 15 pounds, he had passed his work physical with "flying colors" for the first time ever, and he was down to one blood pressure medication, AND his cardiologist was considering taking him off of that one as well. We discussed options for the remaining lead he had stored, and he decided to continue with another 3 months of chelation.

After another 4 months, Jerry came back and was off of blood pressure medications with a very well controlled blood pressure. His lead only went down to 3.5 (we rarely see people get to zero, as there seems to be a law of diminishing returns), and I advised Jerry I thought he had successfully detoxed. He was really happy and now wanted us to look at his gut health as a preventative measure.

He never told his cardiologist what he was doing, because what is customary with many patients is that those who talk to their doctor about Functional Medicine get ridiculed or even fired sometimes. It's a sad state of affairs, but that's the medical world controlled by the pharmaceutical industry.

This is what chelation looked like for Jerry; it was safe and beneficial, and he never had any side effects. When someone successfully chelates like this, I've seen it buy them at least 5 to 10 years of not worrying about metals again (depending on their exposure).

An Alternative to Chelation

My practice has worked with a number of patients who never want to use any medication, it does not matter the situation. And many patients (who have spent considerable time online before coming in to see us) refuse to try chelation. Typically, they've read something bad about it in a social media group or on a blog—and our initial work becomes a matter of educating them about proper chelation. Then, if they are still hesitant, then we discuss its alternatives.

An effective alternative to the use of a chelating agent is modified citrus pectin powder. It is basically a modified nutrient from the skin of citrus fruit. Our intestines can't absorb pectin directly from fruits, but the modified version crosses the gut barrier and gets into the blood, working as a chelating agent.[231] A small study of 5 people showed a 74% reduction in toxic heavy metals without side effects, with the use of PectaSol modified citrus pectin (MCP) (EcoNugenics MCP is the supplement used in this study and the brand that we use).[232] Another study on children between the ages of 5 and 12 showed a dramatic decrease in blood serum levels of lead.[233] These are small studies, so there is still more research to be done, but in my practice I have seen this be an effective alternative. When using MCP, we typically add in some kind of detox support, like you learned about to support phase I and II of detox. My preferred detox support when focusing on heavy metals is called Metalloclear from Metagenics.

Now that you understand more about heavy metals, let's talk about mold.

CHAPTER 8

Mold

Now let's get into one of my favorite topics: mold! Never dreamed I would say those words, but hey, life doesn't always go as planned, right? I'm very lucky that I found Functional Medicine and in turn the world of mold toxicity, because I've been able to help a lot of people using what I have learned. It's worlds apart from the traditional medicine standpoint. To show just how different the traditional and functional views are, consider this: a well-known medical textbook that I used for reference when writing this book is called the *Pathologic Basis of Disease* by Robbins and Cotran. It's over 1,500 large pages, with small writing, too. This book is legendary and terrifying to the medical student. It was fun to go back through now, but guess how many of its pages are about mold toxicity? ZERO. 1,500 pages of scenarios that can go wrong with the human body and only 2 pages about mold—and absolutely nothing on mold toxicity.

When it comes to discussing mold, the most important distinction I need to make is that we are talking distinctly about mold toxicity. The traditional standpoint only focuses on mold allergies caused by mold spores, and this is what the 2 pages in the *PBD* textbook are about. In Functional Medicine, we're talking about mold toxicity caused by mycotoxins. Traditional medical textbooks claim, as they do with the other toxins we've discussed like heavy metals, that we don't know the long-term effects of mycotoxins. This is untrue, I will present a more comprehensive view and evidence to back it up.

What is Mold?

So, what is mold, really? According to the EPA:

Molds are a natural part of the environment and can be found almost anywhere that moisture and oxygen are present. They belong to the kingdom Fungi and live in moist places such as soil, plants and dead or decaying matter. Outdoors, molds play a part in nature by breaking down dead organic matter such as fallen leaves, dead trees and other debris; however, indoors mold growth should be avoided.

When excessive moisture accumulates in buildings or on building materials, mold growth often occurs, particularly if the moisture problem remains undiscovered or unaddressed. Mold growth can occur on:

· Wood   · Foods
· Paper   · Insulation[234]
· Carpet

Mold Spores

Molds spread by producing tiny reproductive cells called spores, which are notably small, ranging in size from 2 to 10 um (less than half the width of human hair). Naturally present in both indoor and outdoor air, spores may remain able to grow and stay problematic for years after they're produced (hence the first thing I learned in Environmental Medicine: the only treatment for a moldy house is to knock it down).

Some call mold nature's recycler, because it feeds on dead and decaying organic material such as trees and plants, also making it not surprising that mold spores often come from farmland, parks, and other places rich in vegetation. Spore counts are higher after extended rainfall or in areas of high humidity. When mold spores settle in a wet area with oxygen, they begin generating thread-like cells called hyphae, which absorb nutrients, allowing mold to grow. Outside mold is good, inside mold is not good—because when hyphae start latching on to wood, carpet, foods, and insulation, it can become a serious problem for the home and its residents.

The Negative Effects of Spores on Humans

According to the Robbins and Cotran textbook, spore inhalation can cause sinusitis, pneumonia, and fungemia (a systemic infection due to mold) in people with a weakened immune system. Traditional medicine says mold affects people with a weakened immune system, whereas in Functional Medicine we are open to the idea that mold may be one of the things weakening the immune system in the first place. Let's take a deeper look at what could cause a weakened immune system:

Traditional

- Genetic abnormalities leading to what are known as Primary Immunodeficiencies. These are people born with a weakened immune system. (It is estimated that there are about 500,000 cases in the United States, with a population of about 329 million, which leaves a 0.001% chance this is the cause of your weakened immune system, but this is the number one thing traditional medicine teaches us on this topic).[235,236]

- Asplenism (not having a spleen)

- Malnutrition

- Chronic infections such as HIV or AIDS

- Autoimmune conditions

- Cancer involving bone marrow

- Iatrogenic (i.e., your doctor did it to you!)
    - Corticosteroids (the types of medications that patients with asthma, autoimmune issues, etc., are put on. Remember learning about cortisol earlier? Well, these are even worse and stronger.)
    - Radiation therapy
    - Chemotherapy

Functional

- Lack of sleep [during sleep, we make more T Cells (killer cells) and improve adaptive immune memory][237]

- Stress (as you learned about in Chapter 2)

- Poor diet [foods high in antioxidants (vegetables and fruits) boost immunity; standard American diet (SAD) suppresses immunity][238]

- Poor gut health (unfunc your gut)

- Environmental toxins like mold

So many differences between the two systems! Now perhaps you can see why it usually involves a struggle to convert one's way of thinking, and perhaps you can appreciate why it is difficult for your traditional doctor to open their mind! And maybe you can see why I chose the route that I did. Which view is more practical for the lay person to grasp conceptually, and then do something about: what is more common, having genetic abnormalities—or eating a poor diet, not getting enough sleep, and being too stressed out?

Traditional medicine says that the person's immune function is more important than the severity of the mold. When we breathe in the spores, they are so small they can get all the way down to the alveoli (remember, that's where gas exchange occurs, and the blood stream is on the other side of the alveoli). Once the spores are in the blood (in the body), the innate and adaptive immune systems will try to eliminate the mold, but if they're weak, the mold invades. The mold, now in the body, releases many different routes of attack, causing protein damage, poor clotting, inhibition of cell protein synthesis, and/ or hypersensitivity reactions, a.k.a. allergies.[239]

If you go to your doctor and say you think you have mold problem, they will test you for a mold allergy and probably tell you, "No, you don't." But that's not necessarily true. What we are here to talk about is mold toxicity. You can have a mold toxicity without being allergic to mold; you can also be allergic to mold but not have a toxicity issue. I think that someone who is allergic to mold will be less likely to have a toxicity because they react to mold exposure and know they're having a reaction. Whereas someone who is just having an issue with mycotoxins is not going to have acute symptoms (as with heavy metals); the toxin will build up slowly because the person does not know they are exposed, leading to eventual disease if left untreated.

Mycotoxins

Mycotoxins are toxic substances produced by mold when mold feels threatened; they are released as a defense mechanism to help mold survive. Not all molds produce mycotoxins, but they are commonly found in buildings that have had water damage,[240] as well as in food, and in cars that have had water damage. Common plants and grain crops where mycotoxins like to hang out include: corn, peanut, wheat, barley, rye, and oat (the staples of the SAD). It has been estimated that about 25% of all crops worldwide are affected by molds.[241] Mycotoxins are heat-tolerant; so they will not be affected by drying and most food and feed processing operations. Mycotoxins can enter our bodies when we breath them in, absorb them through the skin, or when they're eaten, even in microscopic amounts.

The Negative Effects of Mycotoxins on Humans

Disease caused by mycotoxins is called mycotoxicosis; it can present acutely, leading to severe symptom development after only a brief exposure to high doses (I have never seen this; hopefully these patients end up in the ER), or chronically, which is the result of long-term exposure to smaller quantities of the toxin (100% of the patients I have worked with).

Disease can happen through many different mechanisms: mycotoxins inhibit protein synthesis, damage macrophage systems, inhibit particle clearance in the lungs, and increase sensitivity to bacterial endotoxins.[242] Remember, in general, any toxins can cause damage to cells and mitochondria by inducing oxidative stress (inflammation) and generating reactive oxygen species (ROS), activating apoptosis (cell death), inhibiting the electron transport chain (energy production), reducing ATP synthesis (energy), altering membrane permeability, and damaging DNA and proteins. Mycotoxins can affect all organ systems,[243] but individual mycotoxins usually target specific organ systems, including the gastrointestinal, urogenital, vascular, kidney, immune, and nervous system, as well as lead to cancer.[244] One way that I look at mycotoxins differently is not seeing mycotoxins as the sole cause of disease, but as toxins that fill your bucket, contributing to disease. Very rarely does one toxin cause disease; it is a combination of toxins filling your bucket. That being said, in my experience, diseases associated with mycotoxicosis can include:

- Allergies
- Immune system toxicity
- Neurological symptoms
- Cardiovascular symptoms
- Psychiatric symptoms
- Gut issues
- Bleeding
- POTS
- Sinusitis
- Chronic Fatigue
- Hormone disruption
- Cancer
- Mitochondrial dysfunction

Mold mycotoxins cause sympathetic overdrive, which lead to anxiety, rapid heart rate and breathing, hunger, weight gain, and insulin resistance. They also cause vagal dysfunction, which leads to auditory and visual hypersensitivity, trouble swallowing, gut issues, dizziness, and low or high blood pressure. You could argue that anyone who has some or any one of these symptoms with exposure history should get tested. Yet just like with gut issues, heavy metals, and food sensitivities, people with similar levels of mycotoxins can present with totally different symptoms. The symptoms of mycotoxicosis can vary depending on the concentration and length of exposure, as well as age, health, and sex of the exposed individual.[245] I think the hardest part of working with families where we find elevated mycotoxins is that not everyone in the house has symptoms; in my experience, this has been the case over 99% of the time. For example, there could be 5 people living in a moldy house and only one person in the house has symptoms because we all have different buckets and fill them differently. Remember, just because not everyone in the house is sick does not mean that you are not living in a moldy house and that others may not have issues down the road.

According to the EPA, there have been over 200 mycotoxins identified[246] (some studies say over 500),[247] but there are only a few on which most of the research worldwide is done. These are the most common and impactful mycotoxins that we'll discuss. The name of the mold is listed and then the different types of mycotoxins it releases, which we can test for, are listed after.

Aspergillus

Aspergillus is one of the most common molds found indoors and outdoors. It can come from plants, soil, rotting vegetable matter, household dust, building materials, and food. There have been 180 different species of Aspergillus identified. There are 3 toxins we can test for produced by Aspergillus: Aflatoxin, Ochratoxin A, and Gliotoxin.

Aflatoxin

Aflatoxins are some of the leading cancer-causing substances in the environment.[248] Aflatoxin can cause liver damage, cancer, mental impairment, abdominal pain, hemorrhaging, immune system toxicity, coma, and death. It is the most common mycotoxin in a water-damaged building. If you're a pet lover like we are, take note: aflatoxin has been found in many dog foods, as some of the main ingredients of dog food are corn, peanuts, and other grains—the foods highest in aflatoxin. One of the ways they try to get rid of mycotoxins in the feed and food industry is to add mycotoxin binding agents such as bentonite clay to absorb the toxins or enzymes, which deactivate the mycotoxin.[249] But what effects does this have on the nutrients or proteins in these foods? We are often fixing one issue without considering the side effects of the solution.

Ochratoxin A

This is the most common mycotoxin I see come back positive. Ochratoxin A can be especially damaging to the kidneys, immune system, nervous system, as well as multiple effects that cause cell damage, which could affect any system. An interesting study showed that dopamine levels in the brain of mice decreased after exposure to ochratoxin.[250] Some studies have hypothesized that OTA may contribute to the development of neurodegenerative diseases such as Alzheimer's and Parkinson's. Elevated levels are typically due to breathing in toxins in water-damaged buildings. Foods such as cereals, grape juices, dairy, spices, wine, dried vine fruit, and coffee can be higher in Ochratoxin A. One of my favorite routes of detox is through using infrared sauna. Studies have found Ochratoxin A in sweat.[251] (More to come on detox soon!)

Gliotoxin

Gliotoxion is released by Aspergillus to shut down the host's immune system and allow aspergillus to thrive.[252] Once the immune system is weakened, gliotoxin goes after the nervous system. Gliotoxin elevation is most commonly due to exposure to water-damaged buildings or from foods which have aspergillus.

Penicillium

You have probably heard of penicillium because we make one of the most famous antibiotics from it, Penicillin. Its discovery and use during World War II saved many lives. It is also found in food, including cheeses like blue cheese and brie, and it is used in sausages and hams to improve taste and block other molds from taking over. But not all penicillium exposure is safe. There are two mycotoxins it can produce which we can test for and should be concerned about:

Sterigmatocystin

Sterigmatocystin is a mycotoxin structurally related to aflatoxin B1, making it also a cancer-causing compound.[253] This is one of the mycotoxins I have never seen elevated, which is a good thing. Sterigmatocystin can be found in different foods such as spices, grains, bread, beer, and cheeses.

Mycophenolic Acid

Mycophenolic Acid is extremely powerful. It's an antifungal, antibacterial, and antiviral. Paradoxically, it is an immunosuppressant, which inhibits the proliferation of B and T lymphocytes,[254] making you more susceptible to infections. It is associated with miscarriage and congenital malformations when the woman is exposed in pregnancy.[255] Here's the craziest thing about mycophenolinic acid: it is a commonly used pharmaceutical drug in patients who undergo organ transplants (the brand names include CellCept and Myfortic). Yes, it is such a strong immune system toxin, it will stop your body from rejecting a new organ, which is amazing for transplant patients, but not amazing for people who get exposed through the environment.

Stachybotrys

Probably the most well-known mold, Stachybotrys is known as black mold. Elevated levels are most commonly due to exposure to water-damaged buildings. There are many different species of Stachybotrys, the most famous being Stachybotrys chartarum because it became associated with "sick building syndrome."[256] There have been outbreaks reported dating back to the 1930s in Europe from this mold. One of the most shocking was infants' lungs bleeding in Cleveland, Ohio, in the 1990's.[257] There are two mycotoxins we can test you for that are produced by Stachybotrys:

Rioridin E

Rioridin E is better known as a trichothecene, a group of over 150 mycotoxins. They are particularly toxic, as they inhibit protein synthesis[258] and induce cell death.[259] They are so strong, there are multiple reports of them being used as biologic warfare agents.[260] Low-level exposure can cause severe neurological damage, immunosuppression, endocrine disruption, cardiovascular problems, and gastrointestinal distress. They are frequently found in buildings with water damage but can also be found in contaminated grain.[261]

Verrucarin A

Verrucarin is another trichothecene mycotoxin also frequently found in buildings with water damage and in contaminated grain. Verrucarin is particularly toxic to the gut, immune system, bone marrow, and spleen. It has a very classic toxic effect, which includes inhibiting protein and DNA synthesis, disrupting mitochondrial function, and causing oxidative stress. The pharmaceutical industry tried to use it as an anti-cancer drug[262] but it was found to be too toxic.[263]

Fusarium

Fusarium can be detected in water-damaged buildings, but is rare, and is commonly found in soil and plants and most famously found in cereal crops, like wheat, barley, and corn.[264] More staples of the Standard American Diet (SAD)!

Enniatin B

Luckily this is another nasty mycotoxin that I rarely see come back positive. It causes damage affecting the biological response of cell defenses, promoting cell damage through inhibition of the cholesterol acyteltransferase and mitochondrial damage.[265] The presence of this mycotoxin makes other mycotoxins more harmful. This goes for most mycotoxins and is particularly a problem because usually if there is water damage in a building, there is more than one mold growing there.

Zearalenone

Zearalenone from Fusarium has been shown to cause liver damage, immune system toxicity, and damage to the blood, and to be pro-estrogenic.[266,267] You learned all about estrogen dominance and the dangers of xeno estrogens earlier.

Chaetomium globosum

Chaetomium globosum has just one toxin we can test for, Chaetoglobosin A. This is another mycotoxin commonly found in water-damaged buildings. It is very common: up to 49% of water-damaged buildings have been found to have Chaetoglo-bosin A.[268] This is especially toxic as it disrupts cellular division and movement, even at very low levels.[269]

Citrinin

Citrinin is a mycotoxin that is produced by many molds, including the same ones as Ochratoxin A. So, fittingly, this is the second most common mycotoxin I see come back positive. Citrinin is mainly found in stored grains, but sometimes also in fruits and other plant products. It is especially toxic to the kidneys[270] and immune system.[271]

Testing

There you have mycotoxins simplified. So, how do we test your body for all these different mycotoxins? In my practice, I have always used Urine Mycotoxin testing from Great Plains Laboratory (GPL). Remember we detox through the urine, so it makes sense to test for toxins in the urine. FYI, GPL uses liquid chromatography mass spectrometry (LC-MS/MS) technology.

According to the laboratory:

"Using this technology, we have a very sensitive test, which is important because mycotoxins can cause serious health issues even in small quantities. Other mycotoxin testing uses ELISA technology, which relies on antibodies. In addition, all the results from urine tests performed at The Great Plains Laboratory are corrected for differences in fluid intake using the technique called creatinine correction. Failure to use creatinine correction can lead to a thirty-fold variation in the concentration of the mycotoxins when there is variation in fluid intake. Utilization of LC-MS/MS technology gives us a precise identification of all our analytes, which prevents having false positive errors. For many of our compounds we can detect amounts in the parts per trillion (ppt) which is about 100-fold better than any other test currently available."

Here is how results present:

	Normal Range
Aspergillus	
Aflatoxin M1	<0.5
Ochratoxin A	<7.5
Gliotoxin	<200
Penicillium	
Sterigmatocystin	<0.4
Mycophenolic Acid	<37.4
Stachybotrys	
Rioridin E	<0.2
Verrucarin A	<1.3
Fusarium	
Enniatin B	<0.3
Zearalenone	<3.2
Chaetomium Globosum	
Chaetoglobosin A	<10
Multiple Mold Species	
Citrinin	<25

Here's a very important point to understand that does not compute with traditional doctors: the level of elevation does not correlate with the level of symptoms. For example, Patient A with an Ochratoxin A level of 20 has many chronic symptoms, whereas Patient B also tests positive with a level of 75 but they feel totally fine. It is not just the lab test that matters, it is the individual; this is where it is crucial to be working with a practitioner who has true experience working with mold toxicity.

Who Should Worry About Mold?

A lot of us! Anybody who currently lives or works or studies in a building that has had water damage and anybody who ever has. Many of us will detox mold on our own once exposure stops, but I've worked with patients who have lived in a brand-new construction for 20 years, and never had water damage, yet when they were growing up lived in the water-damaged basement of their home, and they come back with elevated levels of mycotoxins. We have learned about all the different variables that affect detox, so we can't predict whether you still have mold or not. But if you have exposure history and symptoms, you definitely require mycotoxin testing. I would argue that even if you don't have symptoms, it would make sense to have tests done.

I quickly learned in my career that asking patients if they had been exposed to mold would make me miss the majority of cases. The majority of people have no idea they're even being exposed. It is especially difficult as it is rarely more than one person in the house who has symptoms. To make it worse, the associated diseases can be totally random (e.g., eczema, migraines, autism spectrum, rheumatoid arthritis, lupus, joint pain, fatigue, sinusitis, etc.). It can be anything, so if someone doesn't even know they are being exposed, why would they even think about mold? Their traditional doctor definitely doesn't mention it. If you are worried, search the Institute for Functional Medicine website (ifm.org) and locate a certified practitioner in your area who has experience with mold, keeping in mind that not all will.

Treatment

You may know that I love to use patient stories as an example, so if you want to read an awesome story about mold detox, start on page 20 of *Unfunc Your Gut* with my case study of Abby's acne, allergies, and infertility. The missing piece I'd like to fill in here is exactly what we used to detox Abby from her mold issues.

Step 1: Stop Exposure

This is the number one rule in Environmental Medicine no matter what toxin you're dealing with: before you start "detoxing" someone, make sure the exposure has stopped. If we're trying to detox you from mold but you are breathing it in everyday in your house, we are not going to get anywhere. Doesn't that make sense?

I mentioned earlier that the first thing I learned in Environmental Medicine was that the only treatment for a moldy house is to knock it down. Remember, even once you kill off the mold the spores and mycotoxins can remain for years after. Even dead mold can be an issue. This is another area of controversy. If you talk to a traditional mold remediator, they'll tell you they can get rid of your mold, no problem. I have seen traditional remediation fail over and over again. The worst case was a patient who spent over $200k on remediation over the course of 5 years; despite my warnings to move, he kept having recurring infections and sinusitis issues. He kept finding more mold and finally moved.

There is one company I have referred patients to—The Mold Pros. They service the whole country using more advanced testing and an enzyme/botanical-based mold treatment, which I have seen be successful. FYI, it can be very expensive.

By contrast, your traditional mold inspector will typically measure the amount of spores outside (where they are normal) and compare it to the number of spores inside (not normal to grow). Mycotoxins can be present when spores are not found, so from a toxicity standpoint this testing has no value. My favorite mycotoxin testing of your home is called an EMMA test from RealTime Labs. They send you a kit and you collect small samples of dust typically from the HVAC filter, and you send it back to the lab. The EMMA only tests the 10 most common mycotoxins found, so it's not perfect. I sometimes suggest people use the ERMI test from Mycometrix; this is a DNA/PCR test for 36 different species of mold. This test is also a collection of dust, and we compare the mycotoxins found in your body to the molds or mycotoxins in your home and try to pinpoint your source of exposure.[272]

When it comes to your workspace, I have seen employers be completely unhelpful. They will frequently hire someone who does spore testing and tell you there is no mold. I've had a number of patients order their own ERMI or EMMA testing and come back with positive results. In adults, the type of career I have helped detox the most are schoolteachers, as schools tend to be very moldy and school boards are particularly toxic when it comes to helping with the issue. There are many things about mold exposure that are challenging: moving, quitting jobs, people thinking you're making it up. It can be difficult. But it can also be extremely worth it if you're suffering from unexplained chronic health issues. So first is to test your body, and second is to test your home. I don't have any affiliation with the previously mentioned labs but have found them to be the best in identifying exposure. Remember, you will never detox mold if you are breathing it in every day.

If you find out you have mold in your body and in your home, but remediating or moving are not options, get a HEPA filter with a Merv rating of 13 or 16 and use it for your HVAC system. Think of your HVAC system as the lungs of your home; this filter will help keep the lungs from sending the mycotoxins all over your home. If there are any rooms in the house you spend the most time in, like your office or bedroom, you can get an individual HEPA air filter for that specific room.

Next Steps: What Do You Do Once Exposure Has Stopped?
Sweating

Exercise is a good part of anyone's routine, whether you have mold toxicity or not. What I encourage my moldy patients to do is sauna, usually infrared sauna. Studies have found many different toxins in sweat, including heavy metals, BPA, phthalates, and mycotoxins such as ochratoxin A, as I mentioned earlier. [273, 274, 275]

Why infrared sauna? Infrared saunas should use different types of infrared light, known as far and mid infrared, which should penetrate to the tissues where the inflammation is and where the toxins are stored. They tend to be better tolerated than traditional saunas as they use light (instead of heat) to heat the body in much the same way the sun does. You can get similar effects at a lower temperature, usually between 120 and 140°F compared to the temperature range of a traditional sauna, which can be between 150 and 185° F. When Mackenzie was detoxing from mold, she would exercise and immediately do sauna afterwards and her levels came down in 3 months after her exposure stopped, but it took us 9 months to totally get the mycotoxins out. I strongly recommend to add sauna on top of exercise. I believe that, aside from stopping exposure, infrared sauna is the best way to get mycotoxins out.

Supplements

	Dose	Effects
Glutathione	Use Liposomal Form, my preferred brand is Readisorb, follow instructions on label	• The master antioxidant • Detox Support (phase I and II) • Neuro-protective • DNA, protein, prostaglandin synthesis • DNA repair • Lowers oxidative stress • Vitamins A, C, and E restore glutathione levels[276, 277, 278, 279]
Alpha Lipoic Acid	600mg Twice Daily	• Can counter act effects of mycotoxicosis because of its properties as: • Anti-Inflammatory • Antioxidant • Decreases Reactive Oxygen Species (ROS) • Lowers oxidative stress • Neuro-protective • Increase excretion of toxins[280, 281, 282, 283]
EPA/DHA	2,000mg Twice daily	• Anti-inflammatory • Immunomodulatory effects[284, 285, 286]
Vitamin A	10k IU daily	• Antioxidant • Immunomodulator[287, 288]
Vitamin E	400 IU daily	• Antioxidant • Anti-inflammatory • Immunomodulator[289, 290]
Binders • **Charcoal** • **Clay** • **Chlorella**	Doses vary, I like G.I. Detox from Biobotanical	• Bind toxins in the gut reducing enterohepatic recirculation (reabsorption) • An unfunc'ed gut can also do this[291]
Buffered Vitamin C	Doses Vary, follow instructions on the bottle you are taking, I like Integrative Therapeutics Buffered Vitamin C	• Vitamin C is an Immunomodulator and antioxidant but on its own is very acidic, buffered vitamin C has minerals added, making it more alkaline. • Toxins create acidity which cause cell death, buffered vitamin C can counteract[292]

	Dose	**Effects**
Tri Salts	Doses vary, follow instructions on the bottle you are taking, I like Ecological Formulas Tri-Salts	• Alkalizing minerals, including calcium, magnesium, and potassium have same mechanism of action as above • Be careful some have sodium, which can be an issue depending on your diet and blood pressure

Cholestyramine

This is medication used in traditional medicine for high cholesterol.[293] It works as a bile acid sequestering agent. As we learned in the detox chapter, bile acids in the stool are one of the ways we get rid of toxins, but it is totally normal for them to be reabsorbed. What our bodies weren't prepared for is our toxic environment and all the toxins attached to the bile acids. So it makes sense that something that prevents the reabsorption of bile can help you get rid of toxins. A lot of my patients don't like it because the traditional medicine has 4 grams of sugar per serving and it is taken twice daily. It also has to be taken separately from anything else, which can make figuring out your schedule for the day difficult. But I have seen it be very helpful in aiding the detox of mycotoxins. There is also a tablet form of the same medication called Colesevelam.[294],[295]

Gut Treatment

There are many practitioners in my field who put every patient with elevated mycotoxins on a gut yeast treatment, which involves the use of nystatin, herbs, and probiotics. I typically do not do this unless someone also tests positive for yeast or mold on a stool analysis or Organic Acids Test (see *Unfunc Your Gut* for more information). I have helped many people detox successfully without the addition of this, but I've also seen it be helpful if the person has gut yeast issues.

Diet

There are also many practitioners who suggest to their patients to go on a very strict diet as part of their mycotoxin detoxification plan. It typically involves cutting out moldy foods like all grains, cereals, juices, dairy, wine, coffee, mushrooms, vinegar and foods containing vinegar, breads and other food made with yeast, jarred jams and jellies, sauerkraut, pickled and smoked meats and fish, dried fruits such as dates, prunes, figs, and raisins, soy sauce, hot dogs, sausages, and beef from cows eating contaminated grains. Most of these foods I would not recommend eating anyway, except for coffee, mushrooms, vinegar, and dried fruits. But I have never really seen diet be an influencing factor in someone's ability to detox from airborne mycotoxin exposure. I think these foods are more of a problem in that they can cause an acute toxicity as described above. Some studies found no increase in urine mycotoxins in coffee versus non coffee drinker.[296] However, I typically ask my patients to avoid coffee and other moldy foods for one week prior to their mycotoxin test.

What Should You Do?

If you're worried about mycotoxins, you can find a Functional medicine or alternative doctor to order urine mycotoxin testing for you. If it is positive, the first and most difficult step is to identify and stop exposure. If your test comes back positive, we do not know when the mycotoxins got there. They might be from exposure when you were 5 years old, or you might have mold growing in your attic above your bed. It's possible the test could show previous exposure.

If you test positive, test your home using the EMMA or ERMI tests mentioned earlier, which have you collect dust from your HVAC filter. By testing your living and working place, you can pinpoint whether your positive urine test is due to current or past exposure. Whether to start detoxing if you're still living in the mold is up for debate. Some patients do, whereas some wait until they move away. It is more difficult to detox if you are breathing it in every day.

As far as a detox plan, sauna is my best piece of advice.

Regarding what to do next with medications or supplements, *do not take anything without talking to your doctor first.* Every Functional Medicine patient has a slightly different plan; it is important that you work with an experienced practitioner who can customize a treatment plan for you.

Do not diagnose yourself with mold toxicity using this chapter and life history. Test. Test. Test. In my experience, most patients who have been convinced, by the Internet and other media, that their main underlying issue is elevated mold mycotoxins, test negative. The power of the mind is an incredible thing. Rather than to assume you have mycotoxins, it's better to test first.

And there you have it: some of the science behind mycotoxins, what they are and how they cause disease. So even though your doctor has told you that all your labs are normal, that you're crazy, and to take an antidepressant, the symptoms may not just be coming from your head. This is an introduction to mold and just enough science so you know I'm not just making this up. Having been in the trenches with thousands of patients is where my experience and value lies, and I urge you to take advantage of it for your own well-being.

CHAPTER 9

Household and Environmental Toxins

What other kinds of toxins might you be exposed to? I want to take a look at things that may surprise or shock you. Don't be scared: this next chapter offers insight from Environmental Medicine, including ideas, tips, and solutions for how to clean up your daily environment. Environmental Medicine is a branch of Functional Medicine that helps us address these concerns. Described as the study of interactions between environment and human health, and the role of the environment in causing or mediating disease, it is key knowledge that I've found particularly useful and important for my patients in their healing processes.

Given the number of toxins out there, I am sure you can find more than are mentioned here, and there will probably be more released between the time I write this and when you read it. But in my experience, heavy metal and mycotoxin detox are much higher yield than detox of these other toxins. This means that clinically I have seen life-changing events through the detox of heavy metals, whereas not so much for the household and environmental toxins we are about to discuss. Where I think the significance of these different toxins lies is with how they add to total body toxic burden. Each one that adds up can make it more difficult to get rid of the next one, and on and on we go. And most importantly, it's important to increase awareness. My experience as a recovering addict has taught me that frequently when we learn something about ourselves or our environment, it's hard to un-know that thing. In AA, Step 1 is admitting you have a problem, and the next 11 steps offer a solution. But you can never get to the solution if you didn't know it was a problem in the first place. So first I offer you food for thought and then steps you can take to clean up your environment.

Electric Vehicles/Green Energy

Let's start with something shocking… the Green Energy movement, the focus on renewable energy to reduce carbon in the environment. Sounds amazing and safe, so much so that I bought an electric car thinking I was doing something good. Turns out electric vehicles have *a lot* of side effects. It really reminds me of the glyphosate debate, which we will look at next. The people with all the power and money pushing something on to us that is relatively unknown and that's supposed to make things cleaner and better, but without any thought of the side effects.

Where does toxicity come from due to electric cars? What are the batteries made of? Lithium, known as "white gold." Lithium is mined from the earth, and it's booming. In fact, in the first three months of 2021, U.S. lithium miners raised nearly $3.5 billion from Wall Street investors. [297, 298]

There are two main ways the extraction industry gets lithium out of the Earth: from rock in places like Australia and North Carolina, and from brine in the salt flats in Chile, Argentina, and Bolivia. They also started a massive project in Nevada to get lithium out of clay deposits. Toxic solvents are used and there is mining waste as a byproduct called tailings. [299] This stuff gets into the surrounding water, ground water, streams, and lakes, which means it gets into our bodies, as well as into our plants and animals, so we get even more of it when we eat them.

An interesting story: In May 2016, hundreds of protestors threw dead fish onto the streets in Tibet (China). The dead fish were floating in the Liqi River, along with animal carcasses. Guess what was nearby the river? A lithium mine. This was the third time in seven years! The first time it happened, they had shut the mine down, but reopened and it happened again. Meanwhile, in Argentina and Chile, locals living close to the lithium brining areas have reported contaminated streams used not only by humans and livestock, but also for crop irrigation, along with complaints that the landscape is now covered mountains of discarded salt. These issues may not seem concerning to Americans, but they are, as this is affecting the food you buy and eat. Not to mention the detrimental effects to human beings being displaced from their homes. Research in Nevada found impacts on fish as far as 150 miles downstream from a lithium processing operation.

An even bigger concern is the amount of water used in lithium extraction. In South America, extracting lithium uses approximately 500,000 gallons per ton of lithium. In one region in Chile, lithium mining consumed 65 percent of the region's water. Now, a typical battery from the big electric vehicle car maker uses about 12kg of lithium, and there are 907 kilograms in a ton, so 500,000 gallons of water can produce enough lithium to make about 75 vehicles. It takes around 1 tablespoon of lithium to produce 1 cell phone, meaning, 500,000 gallons of water would make 190,000 cell phones.[300] In Nevada, the biggest lithium project in America is expected to use billions of gallons of ground water, potentially contaminating some of it for 300 years, while leaving behind a giant mound of waste.

To put this issue in perspective, a huge vegan movement followed the release of various documentaries that raised concern over the amount of water used in cattle farming. Because you need 1,847 gallons of water to produce one pound of beef, 500,000 gallons would produce about 270 pounds of beef. So there's not too much difference between beef production, cell phones and cars when it comes to water use, but a lot of the same people that are going vegan to save water are also driving electric cars, and probably completely unconscious of the issues this raises. We're doing our best with the information the government and the big companies, with all their money, give us...

There is also the issue of what to do with the lithium batteries when they are no longer needed. Australian researchers found that only 2% of the country's 3,300 tons of lithium-ion waste was recycled. Lithium batteries degrade over time, and so they can't just be put in a new car. The Birmingham Energy Institute, for example, is using robotics technology developed for nuclear power plants to find ways to safely remove and dismantle potentially explosive lithium batteries from electric cars. These batteries are that toxic.

One last concern, for now, about electric vehicles is that batteries also need cobalt and nickel, commonly found in Africa—and when cobalt comes out of the ground, it is extremely toxic. There have been reports of artisanal mines in Congo where cobalt is extracted from the ground by hand, often using child labor, without protective equipment.[301] According to the CDC, cobalt exposure can harm the eyes, skin, heart, lungs, and may cause cancer.[302] Yikes, I didn't think I would go there, but the more research I did, the more appalling it was.

One more thing to consider is energy from wind turbines. If you've ever taken a road trip through the country, you've seen the fields of endless wind turbines, right? It looks all "clean and green," but have you ever thought about what happens to them when they breakdown or need to be replaced? I'm sorry to have to tell you this, but they are buried in mass graves in states including Wyoming, Iowa, and South Dakota. A patient I worked with who grew up in Wyoming told me about seeing the massive landfills full of these blades. One blade can be longer than a Boeing 747 wing! These blades were made to withstand hurricane-force winds, so they're very strong and can't be crushed, recycled, or re-used. So when put in their graves, they'll sit there forever. There are some shocking photos if you open the referenced article from Bloomberg News.[303]

Despite all of this, I'm not against green energy, but through the experience of working with patients from a Functional Medicine standpoint, I've learned that you can't always trust the powers that be when they tell you something is safe or clean, when there are huge financial incentives. We have to take charge as individuals and when we do, we can initiate healing waves of change.

Now, I don't know the solution to the energy question, but I don't think we have found it yet. There's a lot of work to be done. I've found this journey of transitioning from a traditional doctor to a Functional Medicine doctor to be jaw dropping so many times, in that I have learned so many amazing things that I would have never believed before. I've found it all so helpful in doing my job of helping people heal that here I wish to share it with you.

Now that we've gotten the shock out of the way, how does this look similar to the glyphosate issue?

Glyphosate

The government and Monsanto—(the maker of Glyphosate, the primary chemical in Roundup™, and the seeds that are resistant to it)—have told the world for years that glyphosate was safe. It took a very long time for them to admit it was harmful. My assumption, based on what you read about electric cars, is the story is going to be the same in time. Glyphosate was introduced into our environment by Monsanto in 1974. In 2020, in one of the biggest settlements ever in the United States, Monsanto was forced to pay more than $10 billion to settle 95,000 claims of cancer and harmful effects.[304] Read those numbers again: $10 billion to 95,000 people. From the beginning, there were reports of concern from the local farmers in countries like India, but there were always articles and "science" discrediting them.[305] I think the significance of the deceit is shown by the fact that one year before the settlement, the United States Government filed a legal brief in support of Monsanto that said the cancer risk "does not exist."[306] The Environmental Protection Agency (EPA) also said that it was a "false claim" to say on product labels that glyphosate caused cancer.[307] When you imagine hearing stories like this over and over, after having spent ten years in the Functional Medicine world, maybe you can understand why sometimes it is hard to "trust the science." What was most shocking was when Michael Taylor was appointed the head of the FDA (United States Food and Drug Administration) after spending time working as Vice President for Public Policy at Monsanto. Can we please *get the func out?!* If you want to learn more about Monsanto, read a book called *Seed Money* by Bartow J. Elmore.

An interesting chart titled "Glyphosate and Autism" accompanied a famous research study published in 2014. The bar graph shows how in 1992, the number of U.S. children ages 6 to 21 with autism showed an exponential climb in the number of diagnoses from the mere thousands in 1992 to over 375,000+ children by 2009. What's just as stunning (and creepy) is that the thin line depicting the proportions of glyphosate and soy applied to corn correlates . . . and climbs up the bar chart *almost exactly.* Although the chart cannot be reprinted here for copyright reasons, I highly recommend you take a look at it—because the picture truly is worth a thousand words:

https://researchgate.net/figure/Correlation-between-children-with-autism-and-glyphosate-applications_fig2_283462716.

Glyphosate was introduced in 1974, so why did it take so long for its use to explode? Glyphosate works by preventing plants from being able to make the proteins they need to survive, so it was too toxic to use broadly. But in 1996, we saw the introduction of genetically modified crops (GMO) that were glyphosate-resistant, so you could spray all the glyphosate you want and the crops would still grow. It started with Roundup Ready soybean, followed a few years later by Roundup Ready cotton and corn, then boom, you see the explosion. What else do you see? Soy and corn, two of the three staples (wheat the other) of the Standard American Diet (SAD). Consider the standard fast-food meal—a burger with fries and soda:

Beef patty: Cows don't live in pastures anymore, they are raised on soy and corn.

Bun: Wheat.

Cheese: Comes from dairy cow fed mostly corn and soy.

Fries: Made of potatoes fried in corn or soybean oil.

Soda: Carbonated water sweetened with high-fructose corn syrup

You can look further into chickens and farm-raised fish, and guess what they're fed? Corn and soy. Those scenarios go on and on.

The chart was staggering—and of course, I'm not at all saying glyphosate causes autism, just showing numbers and coincidences. Important research showed that it's not the glyphosate alone, but the other toxic chemicals found in Round

Up all mixed together, that create a toxic burden.[308] I think this is how Monsanto protected themselves, arguing that glyphosate alone is not so bad, but the combination of the ingredients is deadly. This is essentially the same logic I use when educating patients and audiences: it is not just one toxin that causes disease but your total toxic body burden. Glyphosate, along with its other toxic constituents, causes disease the same way the other toxins cause disease, by causing cell death, but glyphosate is also especially toxic to your immune system, nervous system, reproductive system, and may cause cancer.[309] And it's my belief that our increasingly toxic environment is the reason chronic disease is skyrocketing.

Should you be concerned? I think it's warranted. And we can easily test your body for glyphosate levels in the urine using Great Plains Laboratory. The best things you can do to detox are to:

- Avoid glyphosate by not eating the Standard American Diet, avoid Roundup Ready corn and soy (over 90% of corn and soy in the United States are genetically modified)[310]

- Avoid eating the animals like cows, chicken, and fish which are fed Roundup Ready corn and soy, avoid living in areas where Roundup use is rampant (there are some terrifying studies from farmers in El Salvador, Nicaragua, Costa Rica, India, and Sri Lanka)[311]

- Avoid wearing clothes made with Roundup Ready cotton (yes you can also absorb glyphosate and should consider 'organic' clothes).

Easy right? Don't worry, Chapter 10 will give you some very high-yield ways to get the func out.

Herbicides, Pesticides and Insecticides

Herbicides (weedkillers) are chemicals used to manipulate or control undesirable vegetation (basically kill everything around them *except* what you're trying to grow). Roundup is the most widely used herbicide in America. But maybe the most famous herbicide that you didn't know was an herbicide is Agent Orange. Guess who made the chemical weapon Agent Orange for the government to use in the Vietnam War? Monsanto. I learned this when visiting the Vietnam War Museum in Ho Chi Minh City (Saigon) and could not believe my eyes. How did Agent Orange work? It appears to work by causing uncontrolled cell division in vascular tissue causing people to have darkening of the skin, liver problems and a severe acne-like skin disease called chloracne, along with things like type 2 diabetes, immune system dysfunction, nerve disorders, muscular dysfunction, hormone disruption and heart disease.[312, 313] And these are similar actions to current herbicides still in use…

Next, we have pesticides. They are any substance or mixture of substances intended for preventing, destroying, repelling, or mitigating a pest (can be fungus, bacteria, insects, plant diseases, snails, slugs, and weeds). And insecticides are chemicals used to control insects by killing them or preventing them from engaging in undesirable or destructive behaviors. The most well-known of the insecticides are probably organophosphates, which lead to acetylcholinesterase (AChE) inhibition and accumulation of acetylcholine at neuromuscular junctions, causing rapid twitching of voluntary muscles and eventually paralysis.[314] And this stuff is put into our environment, but don't worry… in "safe" amounts.

There are so many toxic pesticides and insecticides out there, I could not possibly name them all and fortunately I don't have to. As I've stated, I am not worried about just one of these.

I am concerned about your total toxic body burden. Luckily, we can also test for many other specific toxins affecting the food supply, in addition to glyphosate.

Personal Care Products

According to the Environmental Working Group, no other category of consumer products is subject to less government oversight than cosmetics and other personal care products. "Since 2009, 595 cosmetics manufacturers have reported using 88 chemicals, in more than 73,000 products, that have been linked to cancer, birth defects or reproductive harm."[315] American women use an average of 12 personal care products that contain 168 different chemicals. Men use an average of six personal care products that contain 85 different chemicals. As such, what do you suppose are the two biggest concerns?

First, most of these products are applied to your skin—your largest organ! So the chemicals can be absorbed directly into the bloodstream. Even more shockingly, apparently the FDA has allowed the cosmetics companies to regulate themselves. The FDA has little authority to review the chemicals in cosmetics and other personal care products. Personal care products companies do not have to register with the FDA, provide the FDA with ingredient statements, adopt Good Manufacturing Practices, report adverse events to the FDA, or provide the FDA with access to safety records.[316] Get the func out! Some of the most concerning, the majority of which have been banned and replaced with other "safe" chemicals, include formaldehyde, dibutyl, and parabens. In Chapter 10, we cover ways you can decrease your toxic exposure from personal care products.

Everyday Household Materials

What other toxins are lurking around your home? Things that you or your children might be using every day? Growing up, I was not taught to think about what my toys were made of. Or what is on my furniture. Or what I am wrapping my food in. Or what a little device plugged into my bathroom outlet that made it smell good could be releasing in the air. It's not surprising that my family didn't talk about or think about this. My parents were working morning to night so we had food on the table and a roof over our heads. It is surprising to me now that I did go through four years of medical school and three years of residency and no one mentioned toxins. Don't you think? After everything you have been learning?

Everyday household materials include things like your children's toys, pet foods, cleaners, tools, paint, plastic wraps, plastic containers, furniture, sales receipts, gasoline, water bottles, cigarette smoke, air fresheners, glues, memory foam mattresses, PVC pipes, chemicals used for waterproofing or flameproofing your clothes, sunscreen, etc. Some of the types of toxins in these products include: phthalates, pyrethrins, paragons, DDE/DDT, BPA, triclosan, PBDE, PCB's, benzene, styrene, perfluorcarbons, benzophenone-3, vinyl chloride, and trihalomethane.

Here are a few examples of what can happen with exposure to these toxins:

- **Phthalates** have been implicated in reproductive damage, depressed leukocyte function, and cancer. Phthalates have also been found to impede blood coagulation, lower testosterone, and alter sexual development in children.[317, 318]

- **Vinyl chloride exposure** may cause central nervous system depression, nausea, headache, dizziness, liver damage, degenerative bone changes, thrombocytopenia, enlargement of the spleen, and death.[319]

- **High benzene exposure** can cause symptoms of nausea, vomiting, dizziness, lack of coordination, central nervous system depression, and death. It can also cause hematological abnormalities.[320]

- **Pyrethrins exposure** during pregnancy increases the likelihood of autism.[321] They also may affect neurological development, disrupt hormones, induce cancer, and suppress the immune system.[322]

- **Organophosphates exposure** has been associated with things like developing pervasive developmental disorder (PDD), an autism spectrum disorder, and adverse neurologic development.[323, 324]

Now, I'm not worried about just one of these, but I am concerned about how each one adds to your bucket. And again, this is nearly everything in our environment. So what is the best thing you can do? Test your body and clean up your environment. You can reference Chapter 10 for tips.

Testing

My favorite test to assess the extent that these different toxins are contributing to your bucket is also from Great Plains Laboratory (no I don't have any affiliation with them, they are just really ahead of the game, and I have used their tests for a long time). The test is called GPL-TOX Profile (Toxic Non-Metal Chemicals) and it screens for the presence of 173 different toxic chemicals including: organophosphate pesticides, phthalates, benzene, xylene, vinyl chloride, pyrethroid insecticides, acrylamide, perchlorate, diphenyl phosphate, ethylene oxide, acrylonitrile, and more. It is collected as a first morning urine sample and can really be very helpful in assessing your total toxic body burden. I have used this test many times over the years to help objectively show someone what is filling their bucket. Depending on the toxin, we make a treatment plan and monitor the levels as we progress through treatment.

Pharmaceutical Products

These are a different type of toxin, as people take them willingly. Most people have no idea the food they eat, the bottle they drink from, and the deodorant they glide on is adding to their total toxic body burden. Most of the time, these same people are not starting medications because it was their idea; and despite the likelihood of experiencing a number of the side effects rattled off in each commercial, they are being persuaded, "This is the best option for you to feel better."

To keep things simple: there are no drugs you can take that don't come with side effects. Some are worse than others. Now, I am not anti-medication; I think they can be lifesaving and I prescribe medications sometimes. But I think they are clearly being overprescribed without any consideration of why something is happening that would require a medication to correct.

Here is a statistic to back up my claim that they are overprescribed: About 66% of U.S. adults take prescription drugs.[325] We were not born with deficiencies in synthetically made chemical compounds (a.k.a. pharmaceutical drugs). Our bodies are under constant assault by environmental toxins, mixed with a processed diet, and massive amounts of stress. This combination leaves our bodies unable to function properly. The solution is not a pill—the solution is identifying imbalances and correcting them to allow your body to balance itself.

As if things weren't bad enough, in 2020, we added to our buckets when we were persuaded that the only way to be healthy was to isolate and avoid human contact. Did you know that in 2021 there was a 70% increase in fills for Lexapro, 31% increase in Zoloft, and 21% in the generic trazodone.[326] What do those have in common? They are all "anti-depressants." As a recovering addict, I can tell you that when I first tried to get sober, I was put on an antidepressant. I think it did help me, but I was also meditating, praying, doing hours of group therapy every day, individual therapy, AA meetings, and working with others. If I had not been doing all these things, do I think the pill would have helped me? No. Taking anti-depressants can help you in a really difficult time, but they should not be relied upon to fix all your problems and should not be taken long term, in my opinion. As you know, I am a believer that mental, emotional, spiritual health is the most important dimension of health, but it is the most challenging part of getting healthy. What can you do to get off the meds and get healthy? It's easy! Follow the instructions in *Unfunc Your Gut* and *Get the Func Out!*

EMF (Electromagnetic Fields)

EMFs are invisible energy waves that the World Health Organization says are "possibly" carcinogenic to humans.[327] They are emitted by cellphones, microwaves, power lines, Wi-Fi routers, cell towers, computers, fluorescent lights (including CFLs), and other appliances. Reported symptoms include headaches, nausea, fatigue, and loss of libido, anxiety, depression, suicide, conditions like compromised immunity, hormonal dysfunction, and cognitive issues. But the WHO will not acknowledge that they're related to EMF exposure.[328] Why? Maybe because our world would fall apart without these technologies and appliances.

5G

5G is something that has never been used in our environment. I wonder what data will show after 40 years of 5G. Meanwhile, of course we are being told it's totally safe. It employs millimeter waves, a specific part of the radio frequency spectrum between 24GHz and 100GHz, which has a very short wavelength. This section of the spectrum is pretty much unused. Lower frequencies are already heavily congested with TV, radio signals, 4G LTE networks, etc., so they're slower. The use of this new unused wavelength will make your 5G phone even faster. What's the problem? Well, the WHO has already said that EMFs are possible causes of cancer, and separate studies have shown short-term exposure to millimeter waves can have adverse physiological effects in the peripheral nervous system, the immune system, and the cardiovascular system.[329] Should we trust the science, when it's being argued that the available studies[330] do not provide adequate and sufficient information for a meaningful safety assessment? Despite all this information, 5G has been rapidly pushed through. Kind of like glyphosate and electric cars. Time will tell. But you don't have to wait. In fact, you can feel it when you come back into an electromagnetic field after being in nature for a while.

In the meantime, check out Chapter 10 for suggestions on how to guard yourself against EMF exposure.

It's all pretty shocking right?

The more I learned about Environmental Medicine, the more stunned I was. But at some point, I hit a saturation point where it does not surprise me what lengths the corporations making the big money, and the politicians they influence, will go to protect their money and power with total lack of regard for the average person. Thankfully, your health is in your control, and you can take steps to protect yourself.

CHAPTER 10

Get the Func Out

To finish things off, we are going to talk about how you get the func out. First, you learned about balancing your hormones, and then you learned about how to get rid of heavy metals and mycotoxins. These are all things that I recommend you find a doctor you trust and who has sufficient experience to assist you with these kinds of issues. I am going to mention a few supplements, but please do not buy or begin taking any supplements without consulting to your doctor first.

Now let's consider, who should be *getting the func out?*

Anyone alive in the 2020s, and especially if you have any of these symptoms:

- Loss of chemical tolerance
- Intolerance to smells
- Intolerance to jewelry
- Intolerance to shampoo, lotions, detergents
- Food sensitivities
- Constant skin outbreaks
- Constant allergies
- Fatigue
- Muscle aches
- Joint pain
- Sinus congestion
- Postnasal drip
- Headaches
- Gas/Bloating
- Constipation
- Diarrhea
- Foul-smelling stools
- Heartburn
- Hormonal imbalances
- Insomnia
- Difficulty concentrating

- Food cravings
- Water retention
- Trouble losing weight
- Skin problems like rashes, eczema, psoriasis, acne
- Canker sores
- Dark circles under the eyes
- Premenstrual syndrome
- Bad breath
- EMF sensitivity

Any of these sound familiar? Most, if not all, of us will be dealing with any number of these symptoms at various points in life, depending on how loaded "our buckets" are with toxins at any given time. The following tips are not in any specific order, but they are high-yield considerations. Remember, the first step in any kind of detox is to stop exposure, so that is our predominant focus.

Mental, Emotional and Spiritual Health

When you're stressed, nothing seems to work properly. Stressed bodies develop low stomach acid and leaky gut, which allows more toxins into the body, putting a strain on the liver and kidneys. If suffering in these ways, you'll be less motivated to exercise so you won't sweat enough, and you will weaken your immune system, making it more difficult to fend off toxins. At this rate, a person risks never *getting the func out* of their hormones, their cortisol will remain high, their reproductive hormones will be imbalanced, their thyroid will not work as well, and their insulin will rise. Yet there is NOTHING more important to your health than your mental, emotional and spiritual health.

You can follow ALL the upcoming tips, take supplements, and follow a strict diet, but your health will not budge if you don't increase spiritual awareness. Your sympathetic nervous system is activated by stress and puts you in the "fight or flight" response, constantly. Relaxation puts you into the parasympathetic response, which opens up the lymphatic system, the blood vessels, the liver, the gallbladder, the skin, the kidneys and the lungs, and allows your gut to function properly in order for you to *get the func out* (detoxify). It is so essential, I will say it again: there is nothing more important for your hormones or detoxing than your mental, emotional, spiritual health. Reference Chapter 2 and my first book, *Unfunc Your Gut*, for strategies to improve your mental, emotional, and spiritual health.

Sleep

During sleep, your body regenerates. The way I look at it is: we are under attack all day long, and sleep is when your immune system restores, preparing you to fight again the next day. Studies even showed that your brain detoxes at night, pushing toxins out.[331] In America, they estimate 50 to 70 million people suffer with sleep problems; so if you're one of them, here are some simple tips to help out:

- Go to bed before 11pm

- Try not to nap during the day (max 45 minutes if you do)

- Don't watch TV in bed, especially the news (your bed should be for 2 things)

- Take baths with Epsom salts

- Try a side-sleeper pillow if you sleep on your side

- Put a body pillow between your knees to align your back and shoulders

- Avoid eating and alcohol within 3 hours of bed

- Don't check your email within 3 hours of bedtime

- Cover your eyes or use dark shades if light wakes you up

- Avoid caffeine after 2pm

- Don't open your credit card or bank account statements before bed

- Try not to argue, and if you do, resolve it before bedtime

- Be nice to yourself and avoid negative judgments about not being able to sleep

- Go over your med list with your doctor (for example, I've met patients who were taking their thyroid medicine before bed and it was activating their systems; please go back to Chapter 1 and review all the functions of the thyroid to understand why)

- Don't work out after 6pm

- Write in a journal

- Meditate when you wake up and just before bed, but stay alert (there are guided meditations that can be used specifically before bed to help you sleep deeper)

Supplements for Sleep

Note: These are taken 30 to 60 minutes before bed.

Cortisol Manager (Integrative Therapeutics)	1-2 tablets
Night Rest (Source Naturals)	1-2 tablets
Melatonin (to fall asleep)	1-5mg
Melatonin SR (sustained release, to stay asleep)	5-20mg
5-HTP	100-200mg
Taurine	500-2,000mg
Magnesium Glycinate	450mg

Don't take all of these, just try one at a time—and only after going over each option with your doctor first. If you need medications in the short term, make a good plan with your doctor.

Exercise

Exercise looks different for all of us. Benefits of exercise include: increased energy through hypertrophy (growth) of mitochondria, improved insulin sensitivity, increased lean body mass, improved cardiac contractility, decreased blood pressure, improved brain function, increased Growth Hormone release, improved adrenal function, improved immune function, enhanced sleep, up regulated detoxification, improved bone density, improved self-esteem and overall feelings of wellness. I recommend 3 days a week of cardio, complemented by 3 days a week of resistance training, with daily walking (10,000 steps per day) and stretching/flexibility exercises daily. Start with what you can handle and your fitness will improve over time.

Diet

Over 10,000 chemicals are added to food and food packaging materials in the United States.[332] What do you do with your diet?

First, identify food sensitivities! An Elimination Diet is always your first step (explained with 50 delicious recipes in *Unfunc Your Gut*). The Elimination Diet is a short-term process to identify if your body is treating any foods you're eating as a toxin, but a "detox" diet focuses on eating foods which support detox and limit new toxins. So a staple of a detox diet is to eat clean and organic foods. Let's look at some tips:

Eat the Rainbow

- Eat 9 to 12 servings of vegetables and fruit per day

- Buy organic when eating the dirty dozen. The clean 15 vegetables and fruit are OK. (Check the Environmental Working Group website, www.ewg.org, for the list.)

- Buy local, organically grown food to limit pesticides, herbicides, insecticides, GMOs, and heavy metals.

- Eat only grass-fed meat. Also, buy meats in wax paper or freezer wrap.

- Choose only wild caught fish (see a guide to fish below).

- Focus on lean meats over fatty meats (if you eat meat), as toxins are stored in fat.

- Consume cold-pressed oils

- Don't eat canned foods, or plastic-containing foods and liquids just to avoid BPA and other plasticizers. Avoid numbers 3, 6, 7 on plastic; the number 6 on plastic means its releasing styrene gas.

- Avoid plastic lids on your coffee cup.

- Use BPA-free baby bottles.

- Avoid preservatives like BHT, BHA, benzoate, and sulfites.

- Avoid food colorings FD&C yellow #5, #6.

- Avoid artificial sweeteners like sucralose and aspartame.

- Cook with non-toxic pans, skillets, and undamaged pots.

- Choose alternatives to nonstick cookware: stainless steel, cast iron, ceramic titanium, porcelain enameled iron, and anodized aluminum.

- Don't use crystal glasses, as they may contain toxic levels of lead and cadmium.

- Never microwave food or liquids in a plastic container or plastic cling wrap. If you microwave, use glass or ceramic containers instead.

- Store food and liquids in stainless steel, porcelain, Pyrex or glass instead.

- Bring your own mug when buying coffee.

- Drink pure water! Half your body weight in ounces (180 pounds = 90 oz.) of water daily.

- Cut out foods with added sugar. If you need a sweetener, use a small amount of brown rice syrup, stevia, honey, maple syrup, fruit concentrates, monk fruit, or ripe fruit.

- Incorporate intermittent fasting into your lifestyle.

Protein

Protein is an underrated detox food and it should be eaten with every meal. You need the amino acids from protein to bind the toxins that have gone through Phase I and II of detox so they can be carried out of the body. Protein also stabilizes blood sugar (think of what you learned in Chapter 3 and how important it is to stabilize your blood sugars). Vegetable or meat protein is OK. You know what a great vegetarian protein is? Soy. Soy is great for phase I and II of detox due to isoflavones, and a high-quality soy can actually improve estrogen metabolism.

One piece of bad news is that you should avoid shellfish. They tend to accumulate a lot of the toxins in the oceans, seas, lakes, and rivers. Which fish are OK? Here is a guide to mercury in fish:

Highest Mercury DON'T EAT	King Mackerel, Marlin, Orange Roughy, Shark, Swordfish, Tilefish, Tuna (Bigeye, Ahi)
High Mercury (3 Servings or less per month)	Bluefish Grouper, Mackerel (Spanish, Gulf), Chilean Sea Bass, Canned Albacore Tuna, Yellowfin Tuna
Moderate Mercury (6 servings or less per month)	Bass (Striped, Black), Carp, Alaskan Cod, White Pacific Croaker, Atlantic Halibut, Pacific Halibut, Jacksmelt, Lobster, Mahi Mahi, Monkfish, Perch, Sablefish, Skate, Snapper, Canned chunk light Tuna, Skipjack Tuna, Sea Trout
Least Mercury (No maximum)	Anchovies, Butterfish, Catfish, Crawfish, Atlantic Croaker, Flounder, Atlantic Haddock, Hake, Herring, Mackerel (N. Atlantic, Chub), Mullet, Oyster, Ocean Perch, Plaice, Pollock, Canned & Fresh Salmon, Sardine, Shad, Sole, Squid, Calamari, Tilapia, Freshwater Trout, Whitefish, Whiting

Fats and Oils

Avocado, coconut, ghee, extra virgin olive, flaxseed, rice bran, hempseed, and sesame seed oils are the preferred oils for detoxification. Look for minimally refined, cold-pressed, organic, non-GMO oils that are not in plastic bottles. If oil becomes rancid it actually makes it toxic. Store oils in a dark place.

We looked at foods high in antioxidants in Chapter 7, so now let's look at foods that support Phase I and II of detox.

Phase I	
Glutathione	Asparagus, curcumin, broccoli, avocado, spinach, garlic, whey protein. Foods that support glutathione; foods high in vitamin C, selenium, and cysteine-rich foods: Duck, egg yolk, whey protein, red pepper, garlic, onion, broccoli, Brussels sprouts, gluten-free oats, sprouted lentils
Cobalamin (B12)	Sardines, salmon, tuna, cod, lamb, beef
Folic Acid (B9)	Lentils, pinto beans, garbanzo beans, black beans, navy beans, turnip greens, broccoli
Pyrodoxine (B6)	Tuna, turkey, beef, chicken, salmon, sweet potato, potato, sunflower seeds, spinach, banana
Niacin (B3)	Tuna, chicken, turkey, salmon, lamb, beef, sardines, brown rice
Riboflavin (B2)	Soybeans, spinach, tempeh, crimini mushrooms, eggs, asparagus, almonds, turkey
Branched chain amino acids	Chicken, fish, eggs, whey protein
Flavonoids	See above
Phospholipids	Soy, sunflower seeds, eggs
Phase II	
Glutathione	See Above

Phase II	
Glucuronidation	Plant fibers
	Turmeric (curcumin)
	Foods high in alpha and beta-carotene: Pumpkins, carrots, squash, sweet potatoes, collards, red peppers, spinach, mustard greens, chard, dandelion greens, cantaloupe, romaine lettuce
	Food high in quercetin: Apples, onion, kale, cherries, red wine, extra virgin olive oil, beans, broccoli, tea
	Foods high in chrysin and luteolin: Broccoli, chili peppers, celery, rosemary, honey
	Foods high in D-glucaric-acid: Apples, grapefruit, alfalfa sprouts, broccoli, Brussels sprouts, adzuki beans, tomatoes, cauliflower, mung beans, cherries, apricots, spinach, oranges
	Foods high in magnesium: Halibut, almonds, cashews, soybeans, spinach, oatmeal, potatoes, black-eyed peas, brown rice, lentils, avocados, pinto beans
Sulfation	Chicken, Brazil nuts, haddock, sardine, cod, beef, dried peaches, egg, turkey, almonds, spinach, onion, cabbage, Brussels sprouts, chickpeas, figs, beans/peas, leeks, endive, potatoes
Methylation	Foods high in B12, B9, B6 (as above), and methionine (as below)
N-acetylcysteine (NAC)	Chicken, garlic, cruciferous vegetables
Glutamine	Beef, chicken, fish, eggs, cabbage, beets, beans, spinach, parsley
Glycine	Beef, chicken, lamb
Taurine	Beef, chicken, fish
Methionine	Egg white/whole eggs, sesame seeds, Brazil nuts, soy protein, chicken, tuna, beef, chickpeas, almonds, pinto beans, lentils, brown rice
Cysteine	Beef, chicken, lamb, fish

Now you see why glutathione is called the master antioxidant and why I tell my patients it's the closest thing to a magic pill I have. It actually comes in a liquid, but you get the point. It is the only nutrient that works on Phase I and II of detox. Remember, you need both phases of detox working properly.

Clean Home

We learned about all the different toxins you may be exposed to in your home, let's look at how you can clean it up!

Mold

- If you have ever had water damage to a home or workspace, test your body and your house for mold (see Chapter 8).

Water

- Test your water. I like National Testing Laboratories (https://watercheck.com), where you can test anywhere between 32 to 115 analytes including: disinfectants and their byproducts, heavy metals, inorganic chemicals, physical factors, uranium, volatile organic molecules and trihalomethanes.

- Water filters can be in pitchers, attached to pipes, and installed into your refrigerator. Look for a filter with an absolute rating of 1 micron pore size or smaller.

- Understand different filter types:
  - Carbon-based: Carbon traps and removes contaminants from filtered water; their effectiveness can vary; and they need to be changed frequently but can be a good, affordable option. Look for a carbon filter that has NSF/ANSI 53-certification.

- Ceramic-based: Quality can also vary depending on production; this type can be combined with carbon based.
- Reverse osmosis: These are typically installed directly to your home's plumbing and use pressure to force water through the filter (usually carbon based). These will be more expensive. Reverse osmosis is considered the most effective filter type. They are so effective, they can also remove minerals from the water, so some systems add minerals back in. Look for NSF/ANSI 58-certification.

Dust

- Dust has been found to accumulate SVOC, PVC, vinyl, organophosphates, and pesticides.
  - Focus on your bedroom.
  - Use a HEPA Vacuum frequently (air-sealed unit).
  - Filter air with HEPA/carbon filter.
  - Leave shoes outside (you can spread toxins all over your house that your shoes pick up outside).
  - Remove wall-to-wall carpeting.
  - Make sure your fireplace is airtight.
  - Keep your windows open if you live in an area with good air quality. You can check the air quality index (AQI) of your local area using popular weather apps.

Indoor Air

- Clean your air ducts. Hire someone certified by the National Air Duct Cleaners Association (NADCA), as there are a lot of scams out there.

- Use a high-quality pleated electrostatic air filter and high-quality air purifier. HEPA filters with a MERV rating 7 or higher are great.

Cleaning Products

- Use non-toxic household cleaning products. Make your own. Use https://www.ewg.org as a reference. Lemon juice, essential oils and vinegar are great natural options.

Personal Products

- Commit to using non-toxic personal products. Use https://www.ewg.org/skindeep as a reference. You can lookup sunscreen, skin, hair, nails, makeup, fragrance, oral, and baby products.

- As a general rule, don't wear anything on your body or face that would not be safe for you to eat.

- Stop using antibacterial soaps. Their use has become rampant since 2020, and they used to be loaded with triclosan,[333] but that was banned and has now been replaced with new toxins, which they can argue are safe due to lack of data.

- Try making your deodorant from essential oils.

Dental

- Avoid sodium laurel sulfate (SLS or SLES); it is used as foaming agent in toothpaste

- Watch out for propylene glycol in oral care products.

- Avoid titanium dioxide, used to make toothpaste look white.

- Avoid alcohol-based mouthwashes.

- Avoid Teflon-coated dental floss.

- Too much fluoride can displace iodine in the body; it should only be used topically and not swallowed.

- Avoid bleaching products.

Gardening

- Do you know what great natural weed killer is? Vinegar.[334] And it doesn't come with all the side effects that glyphosate does. Using good judgment, you can look up how to make your own non-toxic pest control applications on YouTube, where you will find many experienced gardeners sharing their great ideas.

Minimize EMF Exposure

- Hire an EMF inspector to give you an evaluation of your home. Use someone certified with experience.

- Paint your walls with EMF paint. One layer of the EMF Paint is sufficient for blocking EMF most of the time. EMF paint usually contains water, graphite, and black carbon.

- Don't carry cell phones against your body, don't sleep with them in the same room, and don't use them in airplanes or elevators.

- Arrange your bed so the head of the bed is not against a wall that is opposite to an appliance that produces electromagnetic radiation like electric panel, electric meter, refrigerator, computer or air conditioner. Don't use an electric blanket. All beds should have less than 0.2 to 0.3 milligauss EMF exposure (your inspector can check or you can test yourself using a gauss meter). Avoid metal frame beds.

- Don't let kids use cellphones or hair dryers.

- Stand 3 feet away from microwaves, toasters, electric stoves, etc., when they're on.

- Plug in your internet instead of using Wi-Fi.

- Don't use electronics like laptop while they're charging.

- Check out a book called *Living Safely with Electromagnetic Radiation* by Jim Waugh.

- It's already happening all over the place, with people leaving cities, like us moving from Chicago to Montana, but consider checking out areas away from lots of electrical sources such as West Texas, Arizona, New Mexico, Colorado, Wyoming, Montana, etc.

Dry Cleaning

- Use eco-friendly dry cleaners. Most cleaners use perchloroethylene (perc), which is a known cancer-causing toxin.

General Tips

- Incorporate 10 minutes of sauna daily.

- Watch out for steam rooms (it was my favorite at my gym in Chicago until I realized they were using the city water to create the steam).

- Take an Epsom salt bath three times per week.

- Try hyperbaric oxygen treatment.

- Practice grounding or electrically reconnecting with the earth.

- Replace vinyl flooring in your home.

- Less toxic choices if choosing plastic products: polyethylene pterephthalate (PETE), high-density polyethylene (HDPE), low-density polyethylene (LDPE), Polypropylene (PP).

- Avoid air fresheners, perfumed candles, and plug-in air fresheners, which off-gas toxic chemicals.

- Avoid handling store receipts that contain BPA.

- Try dry brushing to exfoliate your skin.

- Get a lymphatic drainage massage; it is a form of massage that causes lymph fluids to move around. Your lymphatic system helps remove waste and toxins and circulates twice as much fluid as your cardiovascular system.

- Detox as part of pregnancy planning, as the placenta was designed to carry nutrients not to filter toxins. Researchers found an average of 200 industrial chemicals and pollutants in the umbilical cord.[335]

Travel Tips

- Use personal air filters in rental cars and rooms where you sleep.

- Carry charcoal or clay with you as a binder.

- Hydrate.

- Take your own BPA-free container or mug.

- Opt for a pat-down and avoid the scanner at the airport.

General Detox Foods and Supplements

These are things that have been mentioned throughout the book that support your body's ability to get rid a lot of the toxins we are exposed to. As a physician, I make any supplement decisions with my patients based on their testing. I also use as few supplements for as short as possible, until whatever issue we were working on is gone, confirmed via repeat testing. Most patients expect to come in to my office and walk out with a list of 20 supplements they will now be taking. It is actually the opposite. Most of my patients come in to me already on anywhere from five to twenty or more supplements daily, and I am always supporting people in getting people off of them. Frequently they don't know why they started them and come to the realization that they are clearly not helping, if they are ending up in my office. I think it comes down to social media and the amount of money being put into marketing campaigns that convince people that a supplement will fix them. In reality, it's all about profits, just as with the pharmaceutical industry.

All that being said, I am not against supplements, and I find them very beneficial when used properly. So please do not go out and buy all the things on this list, but find yourself a doctor who can give you a concise plan. Be careful of a practitioner who gives you a long list of things to take without testing or an end game—unfortunately, they are most likely concerned about their profits as well.

	Dosing
Liposomal Glutathione	Doses vary
Swedish bitters	Doses vary
Chlorella	Doses vary
Curcumin	500mg twice daily
Parsley and cilantro	1/2 to 1 cup daily in food
NAC	500 to 1,000g twice daily
Green tea	Doses vary
Quercetin	1,000 to 3,000mg daily
B complex	Doses vary
Sulforaphane	50mg twice daily
Milk thistle (silymarin)	250mg twice daily
Alpha Lipoic Acid	300-600mg twice daily
Calcium D-glucorate	150mg 2 to 3 times daily
Resveratol	150mg twice daily
SAMe	400mg once to twice daily
Glutamine	Doses vary
Glycine	1-3 grams daily

You now have what you need to *get the func out*. This is not a magic 3-day, 10-day or 21-day plan. There are so many of those and they work great, but people usually find themselves back where they were when they're done—whereas in this book, you have tips and habits you can use for a lifestyle change and a lifetime of healthy habits.

There are five main areas I look at with my patients, and the order we proceed in is different in everyone: gut health, diet, hormones and toxins, and mental, emotional and spiritual health. Find a practitioner using IFM.org to search for a certified practitioner, to help you make a plan covering these areas. Readers of *Unfunc Your Gut* learned in depth about diet, gut health and mental emotional spiritual health—and based on the feedback, many who have taken their new insight into their health appointments have up-leveled their digestive health. And now you know how to get your hormones balanced with the steps in Chapters 1 through 5 of this book, along with how to identify and eliminate any toxins you may have accumulated. Remember, the first and most important step is to **stop expo- sure.** And the piece that pulls *everything* together is making your daily focus your mental, emotional, and spiritual health.

ENDNOTES

1   *The pollution in people.* (2016, June 14). Environmental Working Group. Retrieved July 14, 2022, from https://www.ewg.org/research/pollution-people

2   *Exposures add up (survey results)* (2004). Campaign for Safe Cosmetics. Retrieved October 14, 2021, from http://www.cosmeticsdatabase.com/research/exposures.php.

3   Getting To Know Cancer. (2013). *Assessing the carcinogenic potential of low dose exposures to chemical mixtures in the environment.* Retrieved July 14, 2022, from http://www.gettingtoknowcancer.org/taskforce_environment.php

4   Thornton, J. W., McCally, M., & Houlihan, J. (2002). Biomonitoring of industrial pollutants: health and policy implications of the chemical body burden. *Public health reports (Washington, D.C. : 1974), 117*(4), 315–323. https://doi.org/10.1093/phr/117.4.315

5   Cleveland Clinic. (2020, August 14). *How environmental toxins can impact your health.* Retrieved July 14, 2022, from https://health.clevelandclinic.org/how-environmental-toxins-can-impact-your-health/

6   Piazza, M. J., & Urbanetz, A. A. (2019). Environmental toxins and the impact of other endocrine disrupting chemicals in women's reproductive health. *JBRA assisted reproduction, 23*(2), 154–164. https://doi.org/10.5935/1518-0557.20190016

7   Gore, A. C. (2007). *Endocrine-disrupting chemicals: From basic research to clinical practice (Contemporary endocrinology)* (2007th ed.). Humana.

8   O'Connor, J. & Chapin, R. (2003). Critical evaluation of observed adverse effects of endocrine active substances on reproduction and development, the immune system, and the nervous system. *Pure and applied chemistry, 75*(11-12), 2099-2123. https://doi.org/10.1351/pac200375112099

9   Okada, H., et al. (2008). Direct evidence revealing structural elements essential for the high binding ability of bisphenol A to human estrogen-related receptor-gamma. *Environmental health perspectives, 116*(1), 32–38. https://doi.org/10.1289/ehp.10587

10 Chen, X., et al. (2014). Toxicity and estrogenic endocrine disrupting activity of phthalates and their mixtures. *International journal of environmental research and public health, 11*(3), 3156–3168. https://doi.org/10.3390/ijerph110303156

11   Hayes, T. B., et al. (2011). Demasculinization and feminization of male gonads by atrazine: consistent effects across vertebrate classes. *The Journal of steroid biochemistry and molecular biology, 127*(1-2), 64–73. https://doi.org/10.1016/j.jsbmb.2011.03.015

12   US Department of Health and Human Services. (2004, September). *Toxicological profile for polybrominated biphenyls.* Cleveland Clinic. Retrieved July 14, 2022, https://www.atsdr.cdc.gov/ToxProfiles/tp68.pdf

13   Tiemann, U. (2008). In vivo and in vitro effects of the organochlorine pesticides DDT, TCPM, methoxychlor, and lindane on the female reproductive tract of mammals: a review. *Reproductive toxicology (Elmsford, N.Y.), 25*(3), 316–326. https://doi.org/10.1016/j.reprotox.2008.03.002

14   Hallegue, D., et al. (2003, April). Impairment of testicular endocrine and exocrine functions after dieldrin exposure in adult rats. *Polish journal of environmental studies. 12* (5): 557–562.

15   Verhulst, S.L. et al. (2009, January). Intrauterine exposure to environmental pollutants and body mass index during the first 3 years of life. *Environmental health perspectives. 117*(1): 122–6. doi:10.1289/ehp.0800003. PMC 2627855. PMID 19165398.

16   Doumouchtsis, K. K., et al. (2009). The effect of lead intoxication on endocrine functions. *Journal of endocrinological investigation, 32*(2), 175–183. https://doi.org/10.1007/BF03345710

17   Bader, W. (2011). *Sleep safe in a toxic world (2nd edition).* Freedom Press.

18   Lin, C. C., et al. (2013). Exposure to multiple low-level chemicals in relation to reproductive hormones in premenopausal women involved in liquid crystal display manufacture. *International journal of environmental research and public health, 10*(4), 1406–1417. https://doi.org/10.3390/ijerph10041406

19   Ahlbom, A., et al. (2000). A pooled analysis of magnetic fields and childhood leukaemia. *British journal of cancer, 83*(5):692-698.

20   Greenland, S., et al. (2000). A pooled analysis of magnetic fields, wire codes, and childhood leukemia. Childhood Leukemia-EMF Study Group. *Epidemiology, 11*(6):624-634.

21   Kheifets L., et al. (2010). Pooled analysis of recent studies on magnetic fields and childhood leukaemia. *British journal of cancer 2010; 103*(7): 1128-1135.

22   Bagheri Hosseinabadi, M., et al. (2019). The effect of chronic exposure to extremely low-frequency electromagnetic fields on sleep quality, stress, depression and anxiety. *Electromagnetic biology and medicine, 38*(1), 96–101. https://doi.org/10.1080/15368378.2018.1545665

23   Kilburn, K. H. (2009). Neurobehavioral and pulmonary impairment in 105 adults with indoor exposure to molds compared to 100 exposed to chemicals. *Toxicology and industrial health*, *25*(9-10), 681–692. https://doi.org/10.1177/0748233709348390

24   Rea, W. J., et al. (2003). Effects of toxic exposure to molds and mycotoxins in building-related illnesses. *Archives of environmental health*, *58*(7), 399–405. https://doi.org/10.1080/00039896.2003.11879140

25   Schneiderman, N., Ironson, G., & Siegel, S. D. (2005). Stress and health: psychological, behavioral, and biological determinants. *Annual review of clinical psychology*, *1*, 607–628. https://doi.org/10.1146/annurev.clinpsy.1.102803.144141

26   Getting To Know Cancer. (2013). *Assessing the carcinogenic potential of low dose exposures to chemical mixtures in the environment*. Retrieved July 14, 2022, from http://www.gettingtoknowcancer.org/taskforce_environment.php

27   Clean Label Project. (2022, April 15). *The best and worst protein powder products*. Retrieved July 14, 2022, from https://cleanlabelproject.org/the-best-worst-protein-powder-products/

28   Lum, G. T. (2010). *Toxic showers and baths*. Citizens Concerned About Chloramine. Retrieved July 14, 2022, from https://chloramine.org/toxicshowersandbaths.htm

29   Lam, J. (2019, January 28). *Alternative toothpaste: How to avoid hidden toxins*. Dr. Lam Coaching. Retrieved July 14, 2022, from https://www.drlamcoaching.com/blog/alternative-toothpaste-how-to-avoid-hidden-toxins/

30   Groch, N. (2021, February 19). *The health hazards of chemical hair straightening treatments*. Living Safe. Retrieved July 14, 2022, from https://livingsafe.com.au/the-health-hazards-of-chemical-hair-straightening-treatments/

31   Sa Liu, S., et al. (2013). Concentrations and potential health risks of metals in lip products. *Environmental Health Perspectives*, *121*(6). https://ehp.niehs.nih.gov/doi/10.1289/ehp.1205518

32   LaMotte, S. C. (2021, June 16). *Makeup may contain potentially toxic chemicals called PFAS, study finds*. CNN. Retrieved July 14, 2022, from https://edition.cnn.com/2021/06/15/health/makeup-toxic-chemicals-wellness/index.html

33   *Dry cleaning chemicals*. (n.d.). Canadian Lung Association. Retrieved July 14, 2022, from https://nb.lung.ca/protect-your-lungs/dry-cleaning-chemicals

34   *Air pollutants*. (n.d.). Centers for Disease Control and Prevention. Retrieved July 14, 2022, from https://www.cdc.gov/air/pollutants.htm

35   Kurtz, T. (2021, March 30). *Eight toxic materials found in common pet products (and how to avoid them)*. Rover.com. Retrieved July 14, 2022, from https://www.rover.com/blog/toxic-pet-toys-beds-safety-guide/

36   Hawkins, M. (2022, February 5). *Mycotoxins in pet food: Know the risks for dogs and cats*. Alltech. Retrieved July 14, 2022, from https://www.alltech. com/blog/mycotoxins-pet-food-know-risks-dogs-and-cats

37   American Thyroid Association. (2019, November 8). *General information/press room*. Retrieved July 14, 2022, from https://www.thyroid.org/ media-main/press-room/

38   American Thyroid Association. (2020, June 8). *Thyroid nodules*. Retrieved July 14, 2022, from https://www.thyroid.org/thyroid-nodules/

39   Arthur, J. R., & Beckett, G. J. (1999). Thyroid function. *British medical bulletin*, 55(3), 658–668. https://doi.org/10.1258/0007142991902538

40   Triggiani, V., et al. (2009). Role of iodine, selenium and other micronutrients in thyroid function and disorders. *Endocrine, metabolic and immune disorders drug targets*, 9(3), 277–294. https://doi. org/10.2174/187153009789044392

41   Farhangi, M. A., et al. (2012). The effect of vitamin A supplementation on thyroid function in premenopausal women. *Journal of the American College of Nutrition*, 31(4), 268–274. https://doi.org/10.1080/07315724. 2012.10720431

42   Kim D. (2017). The Role of Vitamin D in Thyroid Diseases. *International journal of molecular sciences*, 18(9), 1949. https://doi.org/10.3390/ ijms18091949

43   Sategna-Guidetti, C., et al. (2001). Prevalence of thyroid disorders in untreated adult celiac disease patients and effect of gluten withdrawal: an Italian multicenter study. *The American journal of gastroenterology*, 96(3), 751–757. https://doi.org/10.1111/j.1572-0241.2001.03617.x

44   Tsatsoulis, A. (2021, April 8). Stress-Induced th2 shift & thyroid autoimmunity: Unifying hypothesis. *BrainImmune: Trends in neuroendocrine immunology*. Retrieved July 14, 2022, from http://brainimmune.com/the-modifying-role-of-stress-induced-th2-shift-in-the-clinical-expression-of-thyroid-autoimmunity-a-brief-overview-and-unifying-hypothesis/

45   *Hashimoto's disease: Causes, symptoms, diagnosis and treatments*. (n.d.). Cleveland Clinic. Retrieved July 14, 2022, from https://my.clevelandclinic. org/health/diseases/17665-hashimotos-disease

46   *Graves disease.* (n.d.). MedlinePlus. Retrieved July 14, 2022, from https://
      ghr.nlm.nih.gov/genetics/condition/graves-disease/#statistics

47   Saravanan, P., et al. (2002). Psychological well-being in patients on
      'adequate' doses of L- thyroxine: results of a large, controlled community-
      based questionnaire study. *Clinical endocrinology, 5,* 577–585.

48   Wekking, E.M., et al. (2005). Cognitive functioning and well-being in
      euthyroid patients on thyroxine replacement therapy for primary hypo-
      thyroidism. *European journal of endocrinology, 155,* 747–753.

49   Panicker, V., et al. (2009). A paradoxical difference in relationship between
      anxiety, depression and thyroid function in subjects on and not on T4:
      findings from the HUNT study. *Clinical endocrinology, 71,* 574–580

50   Flynn, R. W., et al. (2010). Serum thyroid-stimulating hormone con-
      centration and morbidity from cardiovascular disease and fractures in
      patients on long-term thyroxine therapy. *The Journal of clinical endocri-
      nology and metabolism*, 95(1), 186–193. https://doi.org/10.1210/jc.2009-
      1625

51   Hoang, T. D., et al. (2013). Desiccated thyroid extract compared with
      levothyroxine in the treatment of hypothyroidism: a randomized, dou-
      ble-blind, crossover study. *The Journal of clinical endocrinology and
      metabolism*, 98(5), 1982–1990. https://doi.org/10.1210/jc.2012-4107

52   Gaby, A. R. (2004). Sub-laboratory hypothyroidism and the empirical
      use of Armour thyroid. *Alternative medicine review: a journal of clinical
      therapeutic*, 9(2), 157–179.

53   Neal, D. J. (2021, May 3). *A thyroid medicine's third recall: It's too weak and
      43 had "serious" problems. Miami herald.* Retrieved July 14, 2022, from
      https://www.miamiherald.com/news/health-care/article251108814.html

54   *Acella recalls some levothyroxine tablets due to subpotency.* (2020, Octo-
      ber 7). Healio. https://www.healio.com/news/endocrinology/20201007/
      acella-recalls-some-levothyroxine-tablets-due-to-subpotency

55   Ibid.

56   Brown, N. & Panksepp, J. (2009). Low-dose naltrexone for disease pre-
      vention and quality of life. *Medical hypotheses, 72*(3), 333-337.

57   Cree, B., Kornyeyeva, E., & Goodin, D. (2010). Pilot trial of low-dose
      naltrexone and quality of life in multiple sclerosis. *Annals of neurology,
      68*(2), 145-150.

58   Moore, E.A., et al. (2009) *The promise of low dose naltrexone therapy:
      Potential benefits in cancer, autoimmune, neurological and infectious disor-
      ders.* McFarland Health Topics: Kindle Edition. (Kindle Locations 430-432).

59 Smith, J.P., et al. (2007). Low-dose naltrexone therapy improves active crohn's disease. *The American journal of gastroenterology, 102*(4), 820-8.

60 Ludwig, M. D., et al. (2016). Long-term treatment with low dose naltrexone maintains stable health in patients with multiple sclerosis. *Multiple sclerosis journal – Experimental, translational and clinical, 2*, 2055217316672242. https://doi.org/10.1177/2055217316672242

61 Parkitny, L. & Younger, J. (2017). Reduced pro-inflammatory cytokines after eight weeks of low-dose naltrexone for fibromyalgia. *Biomedicines, 5*(2), 16.

62 McLaughlin, P. J., & Zagon, I. S. (2015). Duration of opioid receptor blockade determines biotherapeutic response. *Biochemical pharmacology, 97*(3), 236–246. https://doi.org/10.1016/j.bcp.2015.06.016

63 Becker, K. (2001). *Principles and practice of endocrinology and metabolism.* 3rd Ed. Philadelphia, PA: Lippincott, Williams, and Wilkins.

64 Talbot, J.A., Kane J.W., & White A. Analytical and clinical aspects of adrenocorticotrophin determination. (2003). *Annals of clinical biochemistry, 40*(5), 453–471. https://doi.org/10.1258/000456303322326371

65 Khorram, O., Vu, L., & Yen, S. S. (1997). Activation of immune function by dehydroepiandrosterone (DHEA) in age-advanced men. *The Journals of gerontology. series A, biological sciences and medical sciences, 52*(1), M1–M7. https://doi.org/10.1093/gerona/52a.1.m1

66 Marx, C. E., et al. (2009). Proof-of-concept trial with the neurosteroid pregnenolone targeting cognitive and negative symptoms in schizophrenia. *Neuropsychopharmacology: Official publication of the American College of Neuropsychopharmacology, 34*(8), 1885–1903. https://doi.org/10.1038/npp.2009.26

67 Hirotsu, C., Tufik, S., & Andersen, M. L. (2015). Interactions between sleep, stress, and metabolism: From physiological to pathological conditions. *Sleep science (Sao Paulo, Brazil), 8*(3), 143–152. https://doi.org/10.1016/j.slsci.2015.09.002

68 Spielman, R. M., Jenkins, W. J., & Lovett, M. D. (2020). Stress, lifestyle, and health. *In Psychology 2e* (pp. 511–548). OpenStax. https://openstax.org/books/psychology-2e/pages/14-1-what-is-stress. Licensed under CC BY 4.0.

69 Bear, T., et al. (2021). The microbiome-gut-brain axis and resilience to developing anxiety or depression under stress. *Microorganisms, 9*(4), 723. https://doi.org/10.3390/microorganisms9040723

70 Guszkowska, M. (2004). [Article in Polish] Wpływ ćwiczeń fizycznych na poziom leku i depresji oraz stany nastroju [Effects of exercise on anxiety, depression and mood]. *Psychiatria Polska, 38*(4), 611–620.

71   Banasik, J., et al. (2011). Effect of Iyengar yoga practice on fatigue and diurnal salivary cortisol concentration in breast cancer survivors. *Journal of the American Academy of Nurse Practitioners, 23*(3), 135–142. https://doi.org/10.1111/j.1745-7599.2010.00573.x

72   Fancourt, D., Williamon, A., Carvalho, L. A., Steptoe, A., Dow, R., & Lewis, I. (2016). Singing modulates mood, stress, cortisol, cytokine and neuropeptide activity in cancer patients and carers. *Ecancermedicalscience, 10*, 631. https://doi.org/10.3332/ecancer.2016.631

73   Tobin, E.T., & Slatcher, R.B. (2016). Religious participation predicts diurnal cortisol profiles 10 years later via lower levels of religious struggle. *Health psychology, 35*(12):1356-1363.

74   Rockliff, H., et al. (2008). A pilot exploration of heart rate variability and salivary cortisol responses to compassion-focused imagery. *Clinical Neuropsychiatry: Journal of Treatment Evaluation, 5*(3), 132–139.

75   Is all this social distancing weakening our immune systems? (2021, November 06). Retrieved December 24, 2021, from https://medical.mit.edu/covid-19-updates/2020/05/all-social-distancing-weakening-our-immune-systems

76   Eisenstein, A. (1957). Effects of dietary factors on production of adrenal steroid hormones. *The American journal of clinical nutrition, 5*(4), 369-76.

77   Jaroenporn, S., et al. (2008). Effects of Pantothenic Acid Supplementation on Adrenal Steroid Secretion from Male Rats. *Biological and Pharmaceutical Bulletin, 31*(6):1205-1208.

78   Platel, K. & Jayalakshmi, S. (2016). Compromised zinc status of experimental rats as a consequence of prolonged iron and calcium supplementation. *Indian Journal of Medical Research, 143*(2):238.

79   Moriguchi, T., Greiner, R. S., & Salem, N., Jr. (2000). Behavioral deficits associated with dietary induction of decreased brain docosahexaenoic acid concentration. Journal of Neurochemistry, 75(6), 2563–2573. https://doi.org/10.1046/j.1471-4159.2000.0752563.x

80   Hutchins, H., & Vega, C. P. (2005). Omega-3 fatty acids: recommendations for therapeutics and prevention. *MedGenMed: Medscape general medicine, 7*(4), 18.

81   Delarue, J., et al. (2003). Fish oil prevents the adrenal activation elicited by mental stress in healthy men. *Diabetes & metabolism, 29*(3), 289–295. https://doi.org/10.1016/s1262-3636(07)70039-3

82   Frederickson, C. J., Suh, S. W., Silva, D., Frederickson, C. J., & Thompson, R. B. (2000). Importance of zinc in the central nervous system: the zinc-containing neuron. *The Journal of nutrition, 130(5S Suppl)*, 1471S–83S. https://doi.org/10.1093/jn/130.5.1471S

83   Prasad, A. S. (2009). Zinc: role in immunity, oxidative stress and chronic inflammation. *Current opinion in clinical nutrition and metabolic care*, 12(6), 646–652. https://doi.org/10.1097/MCO.0b013e3283312956

84   Deans, E. (2013). Zinc: an antidepressant, The essential mineral for resiliency. *Psychology today: evolutionary psychiatry.* 2013, Sept. 5.

85   WHO-FAO. (2001). Human vitamin and mineral requirements. Ch. 16, *Zinc: zinc metabolism and homeostasis.* FAO/WHO-FAO corporate document repository. Retrieved August 29, 2022, from http://www.fao.org/docrep/004/y2809e/y2809e0m.htm

86   Savineau, J. P., Marthan, R., & Dumas de la Roque, E. (2013). Role of DHEA in cardiovascular diseases. *Biochemical pharmacology,* 85(6), 718–726. https://doi.org/10.1016/j.bcp.2012.12.004

87   Hurt, R. T., & Mundi, M. S. (2018). Over-the-Counter Adrenal Supplements: More Than Meets the Eye. *Mayo Clinic proceedings*, 93(3), 276–277. https://doi.org/10.1016/j.mayocp.2018.01.019

88   Panossian, A., & Wikman, G. (2010). Effects of adaptogens on the central nervous system and the molecular mechanisms associated with their stress-protective activity. *Pharmaceuticals*, 3(1), 188–224. MDPI AG. Retrieved from http://dx.doi.org/10.3390/ph3010188

89   Choudhary, D., Bhattacharyya, S., & Joshi, K. (2017). Body weight management in adults under chronic stress through treatment with ashwagandha root extract: a double-blind, randomized, placebo-controlled trial. *Journal of evidence-based complementary and alternative medicine*, 22(1), 96–106. https://doi.org/10.1177/2156587216641830

90   Kuboyama, T., Tohda, C., & Komatsu, K. (2005). Neuritic regeneration and synaptic reconstruction induced by withanolide A. *British journal of pharmacology*, 144(7), 961–971. https://doi.org/10.1038/sj.bjp.0706122

91   Choudhary, M. I., Nawaz, S. A., ul-Haq, Z., Lodhi, M. A., Ghayur, M. N., Jalil, S., Riaz, N., Yousuf, S., Malik, A., Gilani, A. H., & ur-Rahman, A. (2005). Withanolides, a new class of natural cholinesterase inhibitors with calcium antagonistic properties. *Biochemical and biophysical research communications,* 334(1), 276–287. https://doi.org/10.1016/j.bbrc.2005.06.086

92   Kobayashi, K., Nagato, Y., Aoi, N., et al. (1998). Effects of L-theanine on the release of ALPHA-brain waves in human volunteers. *Journal of the Agricultural Chemical Society of Japan, 72*(2):153-157.

93   Nobre, A., Rao, A., & Owen, G. (2008). L-theanine, a natural constituent in tea, and its effect on mental state. *Asia Pacific Journal of Clinical Nutrition, 17 Supplement 1*, 167-8.

94   Kimura, K., Ozeki, M., Juneja, L.R., & Ohira, H. (2007). l-Theanine reduces psychological and physiological stress responses. *Biological psychology, 74*(1):39-45.

95   Ng, Q. X., Venkatanarayanan, N., & Ho, C. Y. (2017). Clinical use of Hypericum perforatum (St John's wort) in depression: A meta-analysis. *Journal of affective disorders,* 210, 211–221. https://doi.org/10.1016/j.jad.2016.12.048

96   Scarpelli, D. G. (1989). Toxicology of the pancreas. *Toxicology and applied pharmacology, 101*(3), 543–554. https://doi.org/10.1016/0041-008x(89)90201-9

97   Halton, T.L., et al. (2006). Potato and french fry consumption and risk of type 2 diabetes in women. *The American journal of clinical nutrition.* 83(2): 284–90. doi:10.1093/ajcn/83.2.284. PMID 16469985.

98   Last, A. R., & Wilson, S. A. (2006). Low-Carbohydrate Diets. *American family physician. 73* (11): 1942–8. PMID 16770923.

99   Stinton, L. M., & Shaffer, E. A. (2012). Epidemiology of gallbladder disease: cholelithiasis and cancer. *Gut and liver, 6*(2), 172–187. https://doi.org/10.5009/gnl.2012.6.2.172

100   Pixley, F., Wilson, D., McPherson, K., & Mann, J. (1985). Effect of vegetarianism on development of gall stones in women. *British medical journal (Clinical research ed.), 291*(6487), 11–12. https://doi.org/10.1136/bmj.291.6487.11

101   Wilcox, G. (2005). Insulin and insulin resistance. *The Clinical biochemist. Reviews, 26*(2), 19–39.

102   ABC News. (2011, February 4). *Worldwide obesity doubled over past three decades.* Retrieved July 14, 2022, from https://abcnews.go.com/Health/global-obesity-rates-doubled-1980/story?id=12833461

103   Centers for Disease Control and Prevention. (2022, May 17). *Obesity is a common, serious, and costly disease.* Retrieved July 14, 2022, from https://www.cdc.gov/obesity/data/adult.html

104   NH DHHS-DPHS – Health Promotion in Motion. (2014, August). How much sugar do you eat? You may be surprised! Retrieved January 12, 2021, from https://www.dhhs.nh.gov/dphs/nhp/documents/sugar.pdf

105   Centers for Disease Control and Prevention. (2022, July 7). *The surprising truth about prediabetes.* Retrieved July 14, 2022, from https://www.cdc.gov/diabetes/library/features/truth-about-prediabetes.html?CDC_AA_refVal=https%3A%2F%2Fwww.cdc.gov%2Ffeatures%2Fdiabetesprevention%2Findex.html

106   Ibid.

107 Hunter, S.J., & Garvey, W.T. (1998). Insulin action and insulin resistance: diseases involving defects in insulin receptors, signal transduction, and the glucose transport effector system. *The American journal of medicine, 105*(4), 331-45.

108 Krauss, R. M., & Siri, P. W. (2004). Metabolic abnormalities: triglyceride and low-density lipoprotein. *Endocrinology and metabolism clinics of North America, 33*(2), 405–415. https://doi.org/10.1016/j.ecl.2004.03.016

109 Watson, G. S., & Craft, S. (2003). The role of insulin resistance in the pathogenesis of Alzheimer's disease: implications for treatment. CNS drugs, *17*(1), 27–45. https://doi.org/10.2165/00023210-200317010-00003

110 Gerozissis, K. (2004). Brain insulin and feeding: a bi-directional communication. *European journal of pharmacology, 490*(1-3), 59–70. https://doi.org/10.1016/j.ejphar.2004.02.044

111 Sechi, L. A., & Bartoli, E. (1996). Molecular mechanisms of insulin resistance in arterial hypertension. *Blood pressure. Supplement, 1*, 47–54.

112 Sharif, E., Rahman, S., Zia, Y., & Rizk, N. M. (2016). The frequency of polycystic ovary syndrome in young reproductive females in Qatar. *International journal of women's health, 9*, 1–10. https://doi.org/10.2147/IJWH.S120027

113 Marshall, J. C., & Dunaif, A. (2012). Should all women with PCOS be treated for insulin resistance?. *Fertility and sterility, 97*(1), 18–22. https://doi.org/10.1016/j.fertnstert.2011.11.036

114 Xu, J., M. D., et al. (2021, July 26). Deaths: Final data for 2019. *National vital statistics reports, 70*(8):1. Retrieved July 14, 2022, from https://www.cdc.gov/nchs/data/nvsr/nvsr70/nvsr70-08-508.pdf

115 UPI. (2021, July 15). *Study: Two in five people in U.S. who died of COVID-19 had diabetes.* Retrieved July 14, 2022, from https://www.upi.com/Health_News/2021/07/15/diabetes-high-risk-condition-death/2781626314320/

116 Riddle, M. C. et al. (2020). COVID-19 in people with diabetes: Urgently needed lessons from early reports. *Diabetes care, 43*(7): 1378–1381. https://doi.org/10.2337/dci20-0024

117 American Diabetes Association. (n.d.). *The cost of diabetes.* Retrieved July 15, 2022, from https://care.diabetesjournals.org/content/43/7/1378

118 American Diabetes Association. (2017). Standards of medical care in diabetes—2017. *Diabetes care. 2017*;40(Suppl 1).

119 DiNicolantonio, J. J., et al. (2017). Postprandial insulin assay as the earliest biomarker for diagnosing pre-diabetes, type 2 diabetes and increased cardiovascular risk. *Open heart, 4*(2), e000656. https://doi.org/10.1136/openhrt-2017-000656

120 Johnson, J. L., et al. (2010). Identifying prediabetes using fasting insulin levels. *Endocrine practice : official journal of the American College of Endocrinology and the American Association of Clinical Endocrinologists, 16*(1), 47–52. https://doi.org/10.4158/EP09031.OR

121 Benson, G. et al. (2011). Rationale for the use of a Mediterranean diet in diabetes management. *Diabetes spectr, 24*(1): 36–40. https://doi.org/10.2337/diaspect.24.1.36

122 Golbidi, S., Badran, M., & Laher, I. (2011). *Diabetes and alpha lipoic Acid. Frontiers in pharmacology, 2,* 69. https://doi.org/10.3389/fphar.2011.00069

123 Yin, J., Ye, J., & Jia, W. (2012). Effects and mechanisms of berberine in diabetes treatment. *Acta pharmaceutica sinica B, 2,* 327-334. https://www.sciencedirect.com/science/article/pii/S2211383512000871

124 Shen, Q., & Pierce, J. D. (2015). Supplementation of coenzyme q10 among patients with type 2 diabetes mellitus. *Healthcare (Basel, Switzerland), 3*(2), 296–309. https://doi.org/10.3390/healthcare3020296

125 Afkhami-Ardekani, M., & Shojaoddiny-Ardekani, A. (2007). Effect of vitamin C on blood glucose, serum lipids & serum insulin in type 2 diabetes patients. *The Indian journal of medical research, 126*(5), 471–474.

126 Ranasinghe, P., et al. (2015). Zinc and diabetes mellitus: understanding molecular mechanisms and clinical implications. *Daru : journal of Faculty of Pharmacy, Tehran University of Medical Sciences, 23*(1), 44. https://doi.org/10.1186/s40199-015-0127-4

127 Karalis D. T. (2019). The Beneficiary Role of Selenium in Type II Diabetes: A Longitudinal Study. *Cureus, 11*(12), e6443. https://doi.org/10.7759/cureus.6443

128 Chen, C., et al. (2017). Association between omega-3 fatty acids consumption and the risk of type 2 diabetes: A meta-analysis of cohort studies. *Journal of diabetes investigation, 8*(4), 480–488. https://doi.org/10.1111/jdi.12614

129 Barbagallo, M., & Dominguez, L. J. (2015). Magnesium and type 2 diabetes. *World journal of diabetes, 6*(10), 1152–1157. https://doi.org/10.4239/wjd.v6.i10.1152

130 Lemieux, P., et al. (2019). Effects of 6-month vitamin D supplementation on insulin sensitivity and secretion: a randomised, placebo-controlled trial. *European journal of endocrinology, 181*(3), 287–299. https://doi.org/10.1530/EJE-19-0156

131 Barber, T. M., Hanson, P., Weickert, M. O., & Franks, S. (2019). Obesity and Polycystic Ovary Syndrome: Implications for Pathogenesis and Novel Management Strategies. *Clinical medicine insights. Reproductive health, 13,* 1179558119874042. https://doi.org/10.1177/1179558119874042

132 Samavat, H., & Kurzer, M. S. (2015). Estrogen metabolism and breast cancer. *Cancer letters*, *356*(2 Pt A), 231–243. https://doi.org/10.1016/j.canlet.2014.04.018

133 Reed, B. G. (2018, August 5). *The normal menstrual cycle and the control of ovulation*. National Library of Medicine: National Center for Biotechnology Information. Retrieved July 15, 2022, from https://www.ncbi.nlm.nih.gov/books/NBK279054/

134 Westervelt, A. (2017, September 20). *Not so pretty: women apply an average of 168 chemicals every day*. The Guardian. Retrieved July 15, 2022, from https://www.theguardian.com/lifeandstyle/2015/apr/30/fda-cosmetics-health-nih-epa-environmental-working-group

135 Stanford Children's Health. (n.d.). *Precocious puberty*. Retrieved July 15, 2022, from https://www.stanfordchildrens.org/en/topic/default?id=precocious-puberty-early-puberty-90-P01973

136 Goodman, S. (2009, December 2). *Tests find more than 200 chemicals in newborn umbilical cord blood. Scientific American*. Retrieved July 15, 2022, from https://www.scientificamerican.com/article/newborn-babies-chemicals-exposure-bpa/

137 Genova Diagnostics. (n.d.). *Hormone test | estrogen metabolism assessment – urine*. Retrieved July 15, 2022, from https://www.gdx.net/product/estrogen-metabolism-assessment-hormone-test-urine

138 Sampson, J. N., et al. (2017). Association of Estrogen Metabolism with Breast Cancer Risk in Different Cohorts of Postmenopausal Women. *Cancer research*, *77*(4), 918–925. https://doi.org/10.1158/0008-5472.CAN-16-1717

139 Muti, P., et al. (2002). Urinary estrogen metabolites and prostate cancer: a case-control study in the United States. *Cancer causes & control : CCC*, *13*(10), 947–955. https://doi.org/10.1023/a:1021986811425

140 Leelawattana R., et al. (2000). The oxidative metabolism of estradiol conditions postmenopausal bone density and bone loss. *J Bone Mineral Res.*, *15*(12): 2513–2520.

141 Napoli, N., et al. (2007). Estrogen metabolism modulates bone density in men. *Calcified tissue international*, *80*(4), 227–232. https://doi.org/10.1007/s00223-007-9014-4

142 Sepkovic, D. W., & Bradlow, H. L. (2009). Estrogen hydroxylation--the good and the bad. *Annals of the New York Academy of Sciences*, *1155*, 57–67. https://doi.org/10.1111/j.1749-6632.2008.03675.x

143 Winer, S. A., & Rapkin, A. J. (2006). Premenstrual disorders: prevalence, etiology and impact. *The Journal of reproductive medicine*, *51*(4 Suppl), 339–347.

144 Gollenberg, A. L., et al. (2010). Perceived stress and severity of perimenstrual symptoms: the BioCycle Study. *Journal of women's health (2002)*, *19*(5), 959–967. https://doi.org/10.1089/jwh.2009.1717

145 Endicott, J., et al. (1999). Is premenstrual dysphoric disorder a distinct clinical entity? *Journal of women's health and gender-based medicine*, *8*(5), 663–679. https://doi.org/10.1089/jwh.1.1999.8.663

146 American College of Obstetricians and Gynecologists. (n.d.). *Premenstrual syndrome (PMS)*. Retrieved July 17, 2022, from https://www.acog.org/womens-health/faqs/premenstrual-syndrome

147 Prentice, R., et al. (1990). Dietary fat reduction and plasma estradiol concentration in healthy postmenopausal women. The Women's Health Trial Study Group. *Journal of the National Cancer Institute*, *82*(2), 129–134. https://doi.org/10.1093/jnci/82.2.129

148 Klein, S., Rister, R., & Riggins, C. (1998). *The complete German commission E Mmonographs: Therapeutic guide to herbal medicines (1st ed.)*. American Botanical Council.

149 Abdi, F., Ozgoli, G., & Rahnemaie, F. S. (2019). A systematic review of the role of vitamin D and calcium in premenstrual syndrome. *Obstetrics & gynecology science, 62*(2), 73–86. https://doi.org/10.5468/ogs.2019.62.2.73

150 Ibid.

151 Gill, J. (2000). The effects of moderate alcohol consumption on female hormone levels and reproductive function. *Alcohol and alcoholism (Oxford, Oxfordshire)*, *35*(5), 417–423. https://doi.org/10.1093/alcalc/35.5.417

152 Woods, N. F., et al. (2014). Endocrine biomarkers and symptom clusters during the menopausal transition and early postmenopause: observations from the Seattle Midlife Women's Health Study. *Menopause, 21*(6), 646–652. https://doi.org/10.1097/GME.0000000000000122

153 NCCIH. (n.d.). Black Cohosh. Retrieved July 18, 2022, from https://www.nccih.nih.gov/health/blackcohosh/ataglance.htm

154 Natural Medicines Database. (2017). Black Cohosh. Retrieved December 24, 2021, from Available at: https://naturalmedicines.therapeuticresearch.com/databases/food,-herbs- supplements/professional.aspx?productid=857#scientificName

155 Woods, N. & Mitchell, E. (2006). Symptoms during the perimenopause: Prevalence, severity, trajectory, and significance in women's lives. *The American journal of medicine. 118 Suppl 12B*. 14-24. 10.1016/j.amjmed.2005.09.031.

156   Bonafide Health. (2021, July 7). *"state of menopause" study to under-
      stand symptoms, treatments and dispositions of menopausal women in
      2021.* Retrieved July 18, 2022, from https://www.prnewswire.com/
      news-releases/bonafide-releases-state-of-menopause-study-to-un-
      derstand-symptoms-treatments--dispositions-of-menopausal-wom-
      en-in-2021-301326568.html

157   Hage, F. G., & Oparil, S. (2013). Ovarian hormones and vascular disease.
      Current opinion in cardiology, 28(4), 411–416. https://doi.org/10.1097/
      HCO.0b013e32836205e7

158   Ustuner E. T. (2013). Cause of androgenic alopecia: crux of the matter.
      Plastic and reconstructive surgery. Global open, 1(7), e64. https://doi.
      org/10.1097/GOX.0000000000000005

159   Clark, B. J., Prough, R. A., & Klinge, C. M. (2018). Mechanisms of Action
      of Dehydroepiandrosterone. *Vitamins and hormones, 108*, 29–73. https://
      doi.org/10.1016/bs.vh.2018.02.003

160   Savineau, J. P., Marthan, R., & Dumas de la Roque, E. (2013). Role of
      DHEA in cardiovascular diseases. *Biochemical pharmacology, 85*(6),
      718–726. https://doi.org/10.1016/j.bcp.2012.12.004

161   Hua, J. T., Hildreth, K. L., & Pelak, V. S. (2016). Effects of testosterone
      therapy on cognitive function in aging: a systematic review. *Cognitive
      and behavioral neurology: official journal of the Society for Behavio-
      ral and Cognitive Neurology, 29*(3), 122–138. https://doi.org/10.1097/
      WNN.0000000000000104

162   Ibid.

163   Griggs, R. C., et al. (1989). Effect of testosterone on muscle mass and
      muscle protein synthesis. *Journal of applied physiology (Bethesda, Md. :
      1985), 66*(1), 498–503. https://doi.org/10.1152/jappl.1989.66.1.498

164   Vingren, J. L., et al. (2010). Testosterone physiology in resistance exer-
      cise and training: the up-stream regulatory elements. *Sports medicine
      (Auckland, N.Z.), 40*(12), 1037–1053. https://doi.org/10.2165/11536910-
      000000000-00000

165   De Pergola G. (2000). The adipose tissue metabolism: role of testosterone
      and dehydroepiandrosterone. *International journal of obesity and related
      metabolic disorders : journal of the International Association for the Study
      of Obesity, 24 Suppl 2*, S59–S63. https://doi.org/10.1038/sj.ijo.0801280

166   Rovira-Llopis, S., et al. (2017). Low testosterone levels are related to
      oxidative stress, mitochondrial dysfunction and altered subclinical
      atherosclerotic markers in type 2 diabetic male patients. *Free radical
      biology & medicine, 108*, 155–162. https://doi.org/10.1016/j.freeradbi-
      omed.2017.03.029

167 Traish, A., et al. (2018). Do androgens modulate the pathophysiological pathways of inflammation? Appraising the contemporary evidence. *Journal of clinical medicine, 7*(12), 549. https://doi.org/10.3390/jcm7120549

168 Lanser, L., et al. (2021). Testosterone deficiency is a risk factor for severe COVID-19. *Frontiers in endocrinology, 12*, 694083. https://doi.org/10.3389/fendo.2021.694083

169 Golds, G., et al. (2017). Male hypogonadism and osteoporosis: the effects, clinical consequences, and treatment of testosterone deficiency in bone health. *International journal of endocrinology, 2017*, 4602129. https://doi.org/10.1155/2017/4602129

170 Goodale, T., et al. (2017). Testosterone and the Heart. *Methodist DeBakey cardiovascular journal, 13*(2), 68–72. https://doi.org/10.14797/mdcj-13-2-68

171 Muraleedharan, V., & Jones, T. H. (2010). Testosterone and the metabolic syndrome. *Therapeutic advances in endocrinology and metabolism, 1*(5), 207–223. https://doi.org/10.1177/2042018810390258

172 Malkin, C. J., Pugh, P. J., Jones, T. H., & Channer, K. S. (2003). Testosterone for secondary prevention in men with ischaemic heart disease?. *QJM: monthly journal of the Association of Physicians, 96*(7), 521–529. https://doi.org/10.1093/qjmed/hcg086

173 de Ronde, W., van der Schouw, Y. T., Muller, M., Grobbee, D. E., Gooren, L. J., Pols, H. A., & de Jong, F. H. (2005). Associations of sex-hormone-binding globulin (SHBG) with non-SHBG-bound levels of testosterone and estradiol in independently living men. *The Journal of clinical endocrinology and metabolism, 90*(1), 157–162. https://doi.org/10.1210/jc.2004-0422

174 Khera, M., et al. (2016). Adult-Onset Hypogonadism. *Mayo Clinic proceedings, 91*(7), 908–926. https://doi.org/10.1016/j.mayocp.2016.04.022

175 Morales, A., & Tenover, J. L. (2002). Androgen deficiency in the aging male: when, who, and how to investigate and treat. *The Urologic clinics of North America, 29*(4), 975–x. https://doi.org/10.1016/s0094-0143(02)00084-8

176 Mogri, M. et al. (2013). Testosterone concentrations in young pubertal and post-pubertal obese males. *Clinical endocrinology, 78*(4), 593–599. doi:10.1111/cen.12018

177 Tremellen, K. (2016). Gut endotoxin leading to a decline in gonadal function (GELDING) – A novel theory for the development of late onset hypogonadism in obese men. *Basic and clinical andrology, 26*, 7. https://doi.org/10.1186/s12610-016-0034-7

178   Aloisi, A., et al. (2011). Hormone replacement therapy in morphine-induced hypogonadic male chronic pain patients. *Reproductive biology and endocrinology, 9*(1):26.

179   Leproult, R. (2011). Effect of 1 week of sleep restriction on testosterone levels in young healthy men. *Jama, 305*(21):2173.

180   Wirth, J. J., & Mijal, R. S. (2010). Adverse effects of low level heavy metal exposure on male reproductive function. *Systems biology in reproductive medicine, 56*(2), 147–167. https://doi.org/10.3109/19396360903582216

181   Johnson, P. I., et al. (2013). Associations between brominated flame retardants in house dust and hormone levels in men. *The science of the total environment, 445-446*, 177–184. https://doi.org/10.1016/j.scitotenv.2012.12.017

182   Wirth, J. J., & Mijal, R. S. (2010). Adverse effects of low level heavy metal exposure on male reproductive function. *Systems biology in reproductive medicine, 56*(2), 147–167. https://doi.org/10.3109/19396360903582216

183   Johnson, P. I., Stapleton, H. M., Mukherjee, B., Hauser, R., & Meeker, J. D. (2013). Associations between brominated flame retardants in house dust and hormone levels in men. *The science of the total environment, 445-446*, 177–184. https://doi.org/10.1016/j.scitotenv.2012.12.017

184   Plessis S.S.D., et al. (2015). Marijuana, phytocannabinoids, the endocannabinoid system, and male fertility. *Journal of assisted reproduction and genetic, 32*(11):1575-1588.

185   Patel, A. S., Leong, J. Y., Ramos, L., & Ramasamy, R. (2019). Testosterone is a contraceptive and should not be used in men who desire fertility. *The world journal of men's health, 37*(1), 45–54. https://doi.org/10.5534/wjmh.180036

186   Prasad, A. S., et al. (1996). Zinc status and serum testosterone levels of healthy adults. *Nutrition, 12*(5), 344–348. https://doi.org/10.1016/s0899-9007(96)80058-x

187   Pokrywka, A., et al. (2014). Insights into supplements with tribulus terrestris used by athletes. *Journal of human kinetics, 41*, 99–105. https://doi.org/10.2478/hukin-2014-0037

188   Mansoori, A., et al. (2020). Effect of fenugreek extract supplement on testosterone levels in male: A meta-analysis of clinical trials. *Phytotherapy research: PTR, 34*(7), 1550–1555. https://doi.org/10.1002/ptr.6627

189   Ibid.

190   Banihani S. A. (2018). Effect of Coenzyme Q10 Supplementation on Testosterone. *Biomolecules, 8*(4), 172. https://doi.org/10.3390/biom8040172

191   Rezaei, N., et al. (2018). Effects of l-carnitine on the follicle-stimulat-
        ing hormone, luteinizing hormone, testosterone, and testicular tissue
        oxidative stress levels in streptozotocin-induced diabetic rats. *Journal of
        evidence-based integrative medicine, 23,* 2515690X18796053. https://doi.
        org/10.1177/2515690X18796053

192   Umeda, F., et al. (1982). Effect of vitamin E on function of pituitary-
        gonadal axis in male rats and human subjects. *Endocrinologia japonica,
        29*(3), 287–292. https://doi.org/10.1507/endocrj1954.29.287

193   Okon, U. A., & Utuk, I. I. (2016). Ascorbic acid treatment elevates follicle
        stimulating hormone and testosterone plasma levels and enhances sperm
        quality in albino Wistar rats. *Nigerian medical journal: Journal of the
        Nigeria Medical Association, 57*(1), 31–36. https://doi.org/10.4103/0300-
        1652.180570

194   Roshanzamir, F., & Safavi, S. M. (2017). The putative effects of D-Aspar-
        tic acid on blood testosterone levels: A systematic review. *International
        journal of reproductive biomedicine, 15*(1), 1–10.

195   Lopresti, A. L., et al. (2019). A randomized, double-blind, placebo-con-
        trolled, crossover study examining the hormonal and vitality effects of
        ashwagandha (withania somnifera) in aging, overweight males. *Amer-
        ican journal of men's health, 13*(2), 1557988319835985. https://doi.
        org/10.1177/1557988319835985

196   Kim, T. H., et al. (2009). Effects of tissue-cultured mountain ginseng
        (Panax ginseng CA Meyer) extract on male patients with erectile dysfunc-
        tion. *Asian journal of andrology, 11*(3), 356–361. https://doi.org/10.1038/
        aja.2008.32

197   Gonzales, G. F., et al. (2002). Effect of Lepidium meyenii (MACA) on
        sexual desire and its absent relationship with serum testosterone levels in
        adult healthy men. *Andrologia, 34*(6), 367–372. https://doi.org/10.1046/
        j.1439-0272.2002.00519.x

198   Scott, A., & Newson, L. (2020). Should we be prescribing testosterone
        to perimenopausal and menopausal women? A guide to prescribing
        testosterone for women in primary care. *The British journal of general
        practice: The Journal of the Royal College of General Practitioners, 70*(693),
        203–204. https://doi.org/10.3399/bjgp20X709265

199   Michaud, J. E., Billups, K. L., & Partin, A. W. (2015). Testosterone and
        prostate cancer: an evidence-based review of pathogenesis and onco-
        logic risk. *Therapeutic advances in urology, 7*(6), 378–387. https://doi.
        org/10.1177/1756287215597633

200   Morello-Frosch, et al. (2009). Toxic ignorance and right-to-know in
        biomonitoring results communication: a survey of scientists and study
        participants. *Environ Health 8,* 6. https://doi.org/10.1186/1476-069X-8-6

201   InformedHealth.org. (2018). *How does the gallbladder work?* Institute for Quality and Efficiency in Health Care (IQWiG). Available from: https://www.ncbi.nlm.nih.gov/books/NBK279386/

202   Hodges, R. E., & Minich, D. M. (2015). Modulation of metabolic detoxification pathways using foods and food-derived components: a scientific review with clinical application. *Journal of nutrition and metabolism, 2015,* 760689. https://doi.org/10.1155/2015/760689

203   LabCE.com. (n.d.). Phase I reactions: Hydrolysis, reduction, and oxidation. *Laboratory continuing education.* Retrieved July 18, 2022, from https://www.labce.com/spg1094049_phase_i_reactions_hydrolysis_reduction_and_oxidati.aspx

204   National Cancer Institute. (2017, December 19). *Harms of cigarette smoking and health benefits of quitting.* Retrieved July 18, 2022, from https://www.cancer.gov/about-cancer/causes-prevention/risk/tobacco/cessation-fact-sheet

205   Kindy, D. (2021, October 14). *Nearly 2,000 Chemicals—Some Potentially Harmful—Found in Vaping Aerosols.* Smithsonian Magazine. Retrieved July 18, 2022, from https://www.smithsonianmag.com/smart-news/nearly-2000-chemicals-some-potentially-harmfulfound-in-vaping-aerosols-180978872/

206   NIH. (2021, October 14). *Statistics and graphs | Division of Cancer Control and Population Sciences (DCCPS).* Retrieved July 18, 2022, from https://cancercontrol.cancer.gov/ocs/statistics

207   CDC's Division of Diabetes Translation. (2017). *Long-term trends in diabetes.* United States Diabetes Surveillance System. Retrieved July 18, 2022, from https://www.cdc.gov/diabetes/statistics/slides/long_term_trends.pdf

208   World Health Organization. (2021, June 9). *Obesity and overweight.* Retrieved July 18, 2022, from https://www.who.int/news-room/fact-sheets/detail/obesity-and-overweight

209   Boat, T.F. & Wu, J.T., editors. (2015). *Mental disorders and disabilities among low-income children.* Washington (DC): National Academies Press (US); 2015 Oct 28. 14, Prevalence of Autism Spectrum Disorder. Available from: https://www.ncbi.nlm.nih.gov/books/NBK332896/

210   Autism Speaks. (n.d.). *Autism statistics and facts.* Retrieved July 18, 2022, from https://www.autismspeaks.org/autism-statistics-asd

211   Tchounwou, P. B., et al. (2012). Heavy metal toxicity and the environment. *Experientia supplementum (2012), 101,* 133–164. https://doi.org/10.1007/978-3-7643-8340-4_6

212   US EPA. (n.d.). *Learn about lead.* Retrieved July 18, 2022, from https://www.epa.gov/lead/learn-about-lead

213 CDC. (2022, July 12). *Facts about hypertension.* Centers for Disease Control and Prevention. Retrieved July 18, 2022, from https://www.cdc.gov/bloodpressure/facts.htm

214 US EPA. (2021, December 21). *Basic information about mercury.* Retrieved July 18, 2022, from https://www.epa.gov/mercury/basic-information-about-mercury

215 Center for Biologics Evaluation and Research. (2018, February 1). *Thimerosal and vaccines.* U.S. Food and Drug Administration. Retrieved July 18, 2022, from https://www.fda.gov/vaccines-blood-biologics/safety-availability-biologics/thimerosal-and-vaccines

216 Ibid.

217 Genchi, G., et al. (2021). Thallium use, toxicity, and detoxification therapy: An overview. *Applied Sciences, 11*(18), 8322. MDPI AG. Retrieved from http://dx.doi.org/10.3390/app11188322

218 KQED. (2016, January 13). *Farms using oilfield wastewater under review for food safety.* Retrieved July 18, 2022, from https://www.kqed.org/science/470114/farms-using-oilfield-wastewater-under-review-for-food-safety

219 Agency for Toxic Substances and Disease Registry. (2007). *Arsenic.* Retrieved July 18, 2022, from https://www.epa.gov/sites/default/files/2014-03/documents/arsenic_toxfaqs_3v.pdf

220 World Health Organization. (2018, February 15). *Arsenic.* Retrieved July 18, 2022, from https://www.who.int/news-room/fact-sheets/detail/arsenic

221 CDC. (2009). *National report on human exposure to environmental chemicals.* Retrieved July 18, 2022, from https://www.cdc.gov/exposurereport/index.html

222 Aldridge, J. E., et al. (2003). Serotonergic systems targeted by developmental exposure to chlorpyrifos: effects during different critical periods. *Environmental health perspectives, 111*(14), 1736–1743. https://doi.org/10.1289/ehp.6489

223 Bradberry, S., & Vale, A. (2009). Dimercaptosuccinic acid (succimer; DMSA) in inorganic lead poisoning. *Clinical toxicology (Philadelphia, Pa.), 47*(7), 617–631. https://doi.org/10.1080/15563650903174828

224 Ruha A. M. (2013). Recommendations for provoked challenge urine testing. *Journal of medical toxicology : official journal of the American College of Medical Toxicology, 9*(4), 318–325. https://doi.org/10.1007/s13181-013-0350-7

225   Hoet, P., Haufroid, V., & Lison, D. (2020). Heavy metal chelation tests: the misleading and hazardous promise. *Archives of toxicology, 94*(8), 2893–2896. https://doi.org/10.1007/s00204-020-02847-7

226   Ibid.

227   Crinnion, W. J. (2009). The benefits of pre- and post-challenge urine heavy metal testing: Part 1. *Alternative medicine review: a journal of clinical therapeutic, 14*(1), 3–8.

228   Walker, J. (2021, December 20). *Biogen cuts price for alzheimer's drug aduhelm by half.* WSJ. Retrieved July 19, 2022, from https://www.wsj.com/articles/biogen-cuts-price-for-alzheimers-drug-aduhelm-by-half-11640001661

229   Milken Institute. (2018, August 28). *The costs of chronic disease in the U.S.* Retrieved July 19, 2022, from https://milkeninstitute.org/report/costs-chronic-disease-us

230   Mayo Clinic. (n.d.). *Succimer (oral route) side effects.* Retrieved July 19, 2022, from https://www.mayoclinic.org/drugs-supplements/succimer-oral-route/side-effects/drg-20066140?p=1

231   Eliaz, I., & Raz, A. (2019). Pleiotropic Effects of Modified Citrus Pectin. *Nutrients, 11*(11), 2619. https://doi.org/10.3390/nu11112619

232   Eliaz, I., Weil, E., & Wilk, B. (2007). Integrative medicine and the role of modified citrus pectin/alginates in heavy metal chelation and detoxification—five case reports. *Forschende komplementarmedizin (2006), 14*(6), 358–364. https://doi.org/10.1159/000109829

233   Zhao, Z. Y., et al. (2008). The role of modified citrus pectin as an effective chelator of lead in children hospitalized with toxic lead levels. *Alternative therapies in health and medicine, 14*(4), 34–38.

234   US EPA. (2022, March 3). *What are molds?* Retrieved July 19, 2022, from https://www.epa.gov/mold/what-are-molds

235   Cooper, M.A, et al. (2003). Primary immunodeficiencies. *American family physician. 2003 Nov;68*(10):2001-2008. PMID: 14655810.

236   Justiz Vaillant, A. A., & Qurie, A. (2021). Immunodeficiency. In *StatPearls.* StatPearls Publishing.

237   Besedovsky, L., et al. (2012). Sleep and immune function. *Pflugers Archiv: European journal of physiology, 463*(1), 121–137. https://doi.org/10.1007/s00424-011-1044-0

238   Childs, C. E., et al. (2019). Diet and immune function. *Nutrients, 11*(8), 1933. https://doi.org/10.3390/nu11081933

239   Barrett J. R. (2005). Liver cancer and aflatoxin: New information from the Kenyan outbreak. *Environmental Health Perspectives, 113*(12), A837–A838.

240   Kuhn, D. M., & Ghannoum, M. A. (2003). Indoor mold, toxigenic fungi, and Stachybotrys chartarum: infectious disease perspective. *Clinical microbiology reviews, 16*(1), 144–172. https://doi.org/10.1128/CMR.16.1.144-172.2003

241   Dodd, C. E. R., Aldsworth, T. G., & Stein, R. A. (2017). *Foodborne Diseases (Food Science and Technology)* (3rd ed.). Academic Press.

242   Godish, T. (2001). *Indoor environmental quality.* Chelsea, Mich: Lewis Publishers. pp. 183–84.

243   Haschek, W. M., et al. (2013). *Haschek and Rousseaux's handbook of toxicologic pathology* (3rd ed.). Academic Press.

244   Schaechter, M. (2009). *Encyclopedia of microbiology.* Elsevier Gezond-heidszorg.

245   Bennett J.W., & Klich, M. (2003). Mycotoxins. *Clin. Microbiol. Rev. 16*(3): 497–516.

246   US EPA. (2022, May 4). *Mold course chapter 1.* Retrieved July 25, 2022, from https://www.epa.gov/mold/mold-course-chapter-1

247   Dodd, C. E. R., Aldsworth, T. G., & Stein, R. A. (2017b). *Foodborne diseases (food science and technology)* (3rd ed.). Academic Press.

248   National Cancer Institute. (2018, December 28). *Aflatoxins.* Retrieved July 19, 2022, from https://www.cancer.gov/about-cancer/causes-prevention/risk/substances/aflatoxins

249   Kabak, B., Dobson, A. D., & Var, I. (2006). Strategies to prevent mycotoxin contamination of food and animal feed: a review. *Critical reviews in food science and nutrition, 46*(8), 593–619. https://doi.org/10.1080/10408390500436185

250   Sava, V., et al. (2006). Can low level exposure to ochratoxin-A cause par-kinsonism?. *Journal of the neurological sciences, 249*(1), 68–75. https://doi.org/10.1016/j.jns.2006.06.006

251   Hope, J., & Hope, B.E. (2012). A review of the diagnosis and treatment of Ochratoxin A inhalational exposure associated with human illness and kidney disease including focal segmental glomerulosclerosis. *Journal of environmental and public health, 2012.*

252   Stanzani, M., et al. (2005). Aspergillus fumigatus suppresses the human cellular immune response via gliotoxin-mediated apoptosis of monocytes. *Blood, 105*(6), 2258–2265. https://doi.org/10.1182/blood-2004-09-3421

253   Díaz Nieto, C. H., et al. (2018). Sterigmatocystin: A mycotoxin to be seriously considered. *Food and chemical toxicology: an international journal published for the British Industrial Biological Research Association*, *118*, 460–470. https://doi.org/10.1016/j.fct.2018.05.057

254   Quéméneur, L., et al. (2003). Differential control of cell cycle, proliferation, and survival of primary T lymphocytes by purine and pyrimidine nucleotides. *Journal of immunology*, *170*(10), 4986–4995. https://doi.org/10.4049/jimmunol.170.10.4986

255   Sifontis, N. M., et al. (2006). Pregnancy outcomes in solid organ transplant recipients with exposure to mycophenolate mofetil or sirolimus. *Transplantation*, *82*(12), 1698–1702. https://doi.org/10.1097/01.tp.0000252683.74584.29

256   Ochmański, W., & Barabasz, W. (2000). Mikrobiologiczne zagrozenia budynków i pomieszczeń mieszakalnych oraz ich wpływ na zdrowie (syndrom chorego budynku) [Microbiological threat from buildings and rooms and its influence on human health (sick building syndrome)]. *Przeglad lekarski*, *57*(7-8), 419–423.

257   Etzel, R. A., et al. (1998). Acute pulmonary hemorrhage in infants associated with exposure to Stachybotrys atra and other fungi. *Archives of pediatrics and adolescent medicine*, *152*(8), 757–762. https://doi.org/10.1001/archpedi.152.8.757

258   Kiessling, K. (1986). Biochemical mechanism of action of mycotoxins (PDF). *Pure and applied chemistry. 58*(2): 327–338.

259   Kaushik, N. K., et al. (2019). Preventing the solid cancer progression via release of anticancer-cytokines in co-culture with cold plasma-stimulated macrophages. *Cancers*, *11*(6), 842. https://doi.org/10.3390/cancers11060842

260   Heyndrickx, A., et al. (1984). Detection of trichothecene mycotoxins (yellow rain) in blood, urine and faeces of Iranian soldiers treated as victims of a gas attack. *Archives belges = Belgisch archief, Suppl*, 143–146.

261   Foroud, N. A., et al. (2019). Trichothecenes in cereal grains: An update. *Toxins*, *11*(11), 634. https://doi.org/10.3390/toxins11110634

262   Liu, Y. B., et al. (2014). Ubiquitin-proteasomal degradation of antiapoptotic survivin facilitates induction of apoptosis in prostate cancer cells by pristimerin. *International journal of oncology*, *45*(4), 1735–1741. https://doi.org/10.3892/ijo.2014.2561

263   Cole, R. J., Schweikert, M. A., & Jarvis, B. B. (2003). *Handbook of secondary fungal metabolites*. Academic.

264 Schrenk, D. (2012). *Chemical contaminants and residues in food (woodhead publishing series in food science, technology and nutrition)* (1st ed.). Woodhead Publishing.

265 Prosperini, A., et al. (2017). A Review of the Mycotoxin Enniatin B. *Frontiers in public health, 5,* 304. https://doi.org/10.3389/fpubh.2017.00304

266 Zinedine, A., et al. (2007). Review on the toxicity, occurrence, metabolism, detoxification, regulations and intake of zearalenone: an oestrogenic mycotoxin. *Food and chemical toxicology: an international journal published for the British Industrial Biological Research Association, 45*(1), 1–18. https://doi.org/10.1016/j.fct.2006.07.030

267 Hueza, I. M., et al. (2014). Zearalenone, an estrogenic mycotoxin, is an immunotoxic compound. *Toxins, 6*(3), 1080–1095. https://doi.org/10.3390/toxins6031080

268 Fogle, M. R., et al. (2007). Growth and mycotoxin production by Chaetomium globosum. *Mycopathologia, 164*(1), 49–56. https://doi.org/10.1007/s11046-007-9023-x

269 Fogle, M. R., et al. (2008). Growth and mycotoxin production by Chaetomium globosum is favored in a neutral pH. *International journal of molecular sciences, 9*(12), 2357–2365. https://doi.org/10.3390/ijms9122357

270 Arai, M., & Hibino, T. (1983). Tumorigenicity of citrinin in male F344 rats. *Cancer letters, 17*(3), 281–287. https://doi.org/10.1016/0304-3835(83)90165-9

271 Liu, B; Chi, J; Hsiao, Y; Tsai, K; Lee, Y; Lin, C; Hsu, S; Yang, S; Lin, T (2010). "The fungal metabolite, citirinin, inhibits lipopolysaccharide/interferon-γ-induced nitric oxide production in glomerular mesangial cells". *International immunopharmacology, 10* (12): 1608–1615. doi:10.1016/j.intimp.2010.09.017.

272 The Mold Pros. (n.d.). *Remediation.* Retrieved July 20, 2022, from https://www.themoldpros.com/services/remediation

273 Sears, M. E., Kerr, K. J., & Bray, R. I. (2012). Arsenic, cadmium, lead, and mercury in sweat: a systematic review. *Journal of environmental and public health, 2012,* 184745. https://doi.org/10.1155/2012/184745

274 Genuis, S. J., Beesoon, S., Lobo, R. A., & Birkholz, D. (2012). Human elimination of phthalate compounds: blood, urine, and sweat (BUS) study. *The scientific world journal, 2012,* 615068. https://doi.org/10.1100/2012/615068

275 Hope J. (2013). A review of the mechanism of injury and treatment approaches for illness resulting from exposure to water-damaged buildings, mold, and mycotoxins. *The scientific world journal, 2013,* 767482. https://doi.org/10.1155/2013/767482

276   Hong S.Y., et al. (2005). Pharmacokinetics of glutathione and its metabolites in normal subjects. *J Korean Med Sci., 20*(5):721-6

277   Martin, H. L., & Teismann, P. (2009). Glutathione--a review on its role and significance in Parkinson's disease. *FASEB journal: official publication of the Federation of American Societies for Experimental Biology, 23*(10), 3263–3272. https://doi.org/10.1096/fj.08-125443

278   Lomaestro, B. M., & Malone, M. (1995). Glutathione in health and disease: pharmacotherapeutic issues. *The Annals of pharmacotherapy, 29*(12), 1263–1273. https://doi.org/10.1177/106002809502901213

279   Alpsoy, L., et al. (2009). The antioxidant effects of vitamin A, C, and E on aflatoxin B1-induced oxidative stress in human lymphocytes. *Toxicology and industrial health, 25*(2), 121–127. https://doi.org/10.1177/0748233709103413

280   Packer, L., et al. (1995). alpha-Lipoic acid as a biological antioxidant. *Free radical biology & medicine, 19*(2), 227–250. https://doi.org/10.1016/0891-5849(95)00017-r

281   Rooney J. P. (2007). The role of thiols, dithiols, nutritional factors and interacting ligands in the toxicology of mercury. *Toxicology, 234*(3), 145–156. https://doi.org/10.1016/j.tox.2007.02.016

282   López-Erauskin, J., et al. Antioxidants halt axonal degeneration in a mouse model of X-adrenoleukodystrophy. *Annals of neurology, 70*(1), 84–92. https://doi.org/10.1002/ana.22363

283   Packer, L., et al. (1995). Alpha-lipoic acid as a biological antioxidant. *Free radical biology & medicine, 19*(2), 227–250. https://doi.org/10.1016/0891-5849(95)00017-r

284   Calder, P. C. (2001). Polyunsaturated fatty acids, inflammation, and immunity. *Lipids, 36*(9), 1007–1024. https://doi.org/10.1007/s11745-001-0812-7

285   Ballantyne, C. M., et al. (2012). Efficacy and safety of eicosapentaenoic acid ethyl ester (AMR101) therapy in statin-treated patients with persistent high triglycerides (from the ANCHOR study). *The American journal of cardiology, 110*(7), 984–992. https://doi.org/10.1016/j.amjcard.2012.05.031

286   Kemen, M., et al. (1995). Early postoperative enteral nutrition with arginine-omega-3 fatty acids and ribonucleic acid-supplemented diet versus placebo in cancer patients: an immunologic evaluation of Impact. *Critical care medicine, 23*(4), 652–659. https://doi.org/10.1097/00003246-199504000-00012

287   Food and Nutrition Board, Institute of Medicine. (2002). Dietary reference intakes for vitamin A, vitamin K, arsenic, boron, chromium, copper, iodine, iron, manganese, molybdenum, nickel, silicon, vanadium, and zinc. Washington, DC: National Academy Press.

288   Palace, V.P., et al. (1999). Antioxidant potentials of vitamin A and carotenoids and their relevance to heart disease. *Free radic biol med., 26*(5-6):746-61. doi: 10.1016/s0891-5849(98)00266-4. PMID: 10218665.

289   Asbaghi, O., et al. (2020). The effect of vitamin E supplementation on selected inflammatory biomarkers in adults: a systematic review and meta-analysis of randomized clinical trials. *Scientific reports, 10*(1), 17234. https://doi.org/10.1038/s41598-020-73741-6

290   *Fryer, M.J. (2000). Vitamin E as a protective antioxidant in progressive renal failure. Nephrology, 5: 1-7.*

291   Hope, J. (2013). A review of the mechanism of injury and treatment approaches for illness resulting from exposure to water-damaged buildings, mold, and mycotoxins. *TheScientificWorldJournal, 2013*, 767482. https://doi.org/10.1155/2013/767482

292   Lee, J. K., et al. (2018). Alleviation of ascorbic acid-induced gastric high acidity by calcium ascorbate *in vitro* and *in vivo*. *The Korean journal of physiology & pharmacology: official journal of the Korean Physiological Society and the Korean Society of Pharmacology, 22*(1), 35–42. https://doi.org/10.4196/kjpp.2018.22.1.35

293   Takenaka, S., et al.. Effects of rice bran fibre and cholestyramine on the faecal excretion of Kanechlor 600 (PCB) in rats. *Xenobiotica. 1991 Mar;21*(3):351-7. doi: 10.3109/00498259109039475. PMID: 1907420.

294   Boylan, J. J., et al. (1978). Cholestyramine: use as a new therapeutic approach for chlordecone (kepone) poisoning. *Science (New York, N.Y.), 199*(4331), 893–895. https://doi.org/10.1126/science.74852

295   Takenaka, S., et al. (1991). Effects of rice bran fibre and cholestyramine on the faecal excretion of Kanechlor 600 (PCB) in rats. *Xenobiotica: The fate of foreign compounds in biological systems, 21*(3), 351–357. https://doi.org/10.3109/00498259109039475

296   Pratt-Hyatt, M., PhD. (2021, August 26). *Common questions with Dr. Pratt-Hyatt: Is there mold in my coffee?* The Mold Pros. Retrieved July 20, 2022, from https://www.themoldpros.com/the-mold-pros-blogs/common-questions-with-dr-pratt-hyatt-is-there-mold-in-my-coffee

297   Penn, I., Lipton, E., & Angotti-Jones, G. (2021, May 7). *Lithium mining projects may not be green friendly. The New York times.* Retrieved July 20, 2022, from https://www.nytimes.com/2021/05/06/business/lithium-mining-race.html

298   McFadden, C. (2021, April 11). *The paradox of "clean" EVs and the "dirty" lithium mining business. Interesting engineering.* Retrieved July 20, 2022, from https://interestingengineering.com/clean-evs-and-dirty-lithium-mining-business

299   Amui, Rachid (February 2020). *Commodities at a glance: Special issue on strategic battery raw materials* (PDF). United Nations Conference on Trade and Development. Retrieved July 20, 2022, from https://unctad.org/webflyer/commodities-glance-special-issue-strategic-battery-raw-materials

300   Xanders, M. (n.d.). *The earthly effects of extracting lithium.* Retrieved July 20, 2022, from https://www.tcc.fl.edu/media/divisions/academic-affairs/academic-enrichment/urc/poster-abstracts/Xanders_Madison_Poster_URS.pdf

301   Niarchos, N. (2021, May 24). *The dark side of congo's cobalt rush.* The New Yorker. Retrieved July 20, 2022, from https://www.newyorker.com/magazine/2021/05/31/the-dark-side-of-congos-cobalt-rush

302   CDC. (n.d.). *Cobalt.* Retrieved July 20, 2022, from https://www.cdc.gov/niosh/topics/cobalt/default.html

303   Martin, C. (2020, February 5). *Wind turbine blades can't be recycled, so they're piling up in landfills. Bloomberg.* https://www.bloomberg.com/news/features/2020-02-05/wind-turbine-blades-can-t-be-recycled-so-they-re-piling-up-in-landfills#xj4y7vzkg

304   Cohen, P. (2020, June 25). *Roundup maker to pay $10 billion to settle cancer suits. The New York times.* Retrieved July 20, 2022, from https://nytimes.com/2020/06/24/business/roundup-settlement-lawsuits.html

305   Andreotti, G., et al. (2018). Glyphosate use and cancer incidence in the agricultural health study. *Journal of the national cancer institute, 110*(5), 509–516. https://doi.org/10.1093/jnci/djx233

306   Cohen, P. (2020b, June 25). *Roundup maker to pay $10 billion to settle cancer suits. The New York times.* Retrieved July 20, 2022, from https://nytimes.com/2020/06/24/business/roundup-settlement-lawsuits.html

307   Ibid.

308   Richard, S., et al. (2005). Differential effects of glyphosate and roundup on human placental cells and aromatase. *Environmental health perspectives, 113*(6), 716–720. https://doi.org/10.1289/ehp.7728

309   Peillex, C., & Pelletier, M. (2020). The impact and toxicity of glyphosate and glyphosate-based herbicides on health and immunity. *Journal of immunotoxicology, 17*(1), 163–174. https://doi.org/10.1080/1547691X.2020.1804492

310 USDA. (n.d.). *USDA ERS—charts of note*. Retrieved July 20, 2022, from https://www.ers.usda.gov/data-products/charts-of-note/charts-of-note/?topicId=a2d1ab41-13b3-48b5-8451-688d73507ff4

311 Guyton, K. Z., et al. (2015). Carcinogenicity of tetrachlorvinphos, parathion, malathion, diazinon, and glyphosate. *The lancet. Oncology*, *16*(5), 490–491. https://doi.org/10.1016/S1470-2045(15)70134-8

312 U.S. Environmental Protection Agency, Office of Prevention, Pesticides and Toxic Substances, Office of Pesticide Programs. (2005). *Reregistration eligibility decision (RED) 2,4-D; EPA 738-R-05-002*. U.S. Government Printing Office: Washington, DC.

313 Vencill, W.K. (2002). *Herbicide handbook, 8th Ed*. Weed Science Society of America: Lawrence, KS. pp. 113-115.

314 US EPA. (2022, May 10). *Insecticides*. Retrieved July 20, 2022, from https://www.epa.gov/caddis-vol2/insecticides

315 Faber, S. (2020, May 5). *The toxic twelve chemicals and contaminants in cosmetics*. Environmental Working Group. Retrieved July 20, 2022, from https://www.ewg.org/the-toxic-twelve-chemicals-and-contaminants-in-cosmetics

316 Faber, S. (2016, September 22). *EWG testimony on exploring current practices in cosmetics development and safety*. Environmental Working Group. Retrieved July 20, 2022, from https://www.ewg.org/news-insights/testimony/ewg-testimony-exploring-current-practices-cosmetics-development-and-safety

317 Xu, S., et al. (2020). Exposure to phthalates impaired neurodevelopment through estrogenic effects and induced DNA damage in neurons. *Aquatic toxicology (Amsterdam, Netherlands)*, *222*, 105469. https://doi.org/10.1016/j.aquatox.2020.105469

318 Chang, W. H., et al. (2015). Phthalates might interfere with testicular function by reducing testosterone and insulin-like factor 3 levels. *Human reproduction (Oxford, England)*, *30*(11), 2658–2670. https://doi.org/10.1093/humrep/dev225

319 CDC Agency for Toxic Substances and Disease Registry. (n.d.). *Vinyl chloride—health effects*. Retrieved July 20, 2022, from https://www.atsdr.cdc.gov/toxprofiles/tp20-c3.pdf

320 USDHHS. (2007, August). *Toxicological profile for benzene*. Retrieved July 20, 2022, from https://www.epa.gov/sites/default/files/2014-03/documents/benzene_toxicological_profile_tp3_3v.pdf

321   Shelton, J. F., et al. (2014). Neurodevelopmental disorders and prenatal residential proximity to agricultural pesticides: the CHARGE study. *Environmental health perspectives*, *122*(10), 1103–1109. https://doi.org/10.1289/ehp.1307044

322   Barrett J. R. (2006). Pyrethroids in the home: Nondietary pesticide exposure in children. *Environmental Health Perspectives*, *114*(9), A544.

323   Furlong, M. A., et al. (2014). Prenatal exposure to organophosphate pesticides and reciprocal social behavior in childhood. *Environment international*, *70*, 125–131. https://doi.org/10.1016/j.envint.2014.05.011

324   Eskenazi, B., et al. (2007). Organophosphate pesticide exposure and neurodevelopment in young Mexican-American children. *Environmental health perspectives*, *115*(5), 792–798. https://doi.org/10.1289/ehp.9828

325   Team, S. (2022, January 21). *Prescription drug statistics 2022*. The Checkup. Retrieved July 20, 2022, from https://www.singlecare.com/blog/news/prescription-drug-statistics/

326   Ibid.

327   National Cancer Institute. (2022, May 30). *Electromagnetic fields and cancer*. Retrieved July 20, 2022, from https://www.cancer.gov/about-cancer/causes-prevention/risk/radiation/electromagnetic-fields-fact-sheet#what-do-expert-organizations-conclude-about-the-cancer-risk-from-emfs

328   WHO. (2016, August 4). *Radiation: Electromagnetic fields*. Retrieved July 20, 2022, from https://www.who.int/news-room/questions-and-answers/item/radiation-electromagnetic-fields

329   Karaboytcheva, M. (2020, March). *Effects of 5G wireless communication on human health*. European Parliamentary Research Service. Retrieved July 21, 2022, from https://www.europarl.europa.eu/RegData/etudes/BRIE/2020/646172/EPRS_BRI%282020%29646172_EN.pdf

330   Simkó, M. & Mattsson, M.O. 5G Wireless Communication and Health Effects—A Pragmatic Review Based on Available Studies Regarding 6 to 100 GHz. *Int J Environ Res Public Health. 2019 Sep 13;16*(18):3406. doi: 10.3390/ijerph16183406. PMID: 31540320; PMCID: PMC6765906.

331   National Institutes of Health (NIH). (2015, September 17). *Brain may flush out toxins during sleep*. Retrieved July 21, 2022, from https://www.nih.gov/news-events/news-releases/brain-may-flush-out-toxins-during-sleep

332 Gordon, M. (2021). *The disproportionate impacts of chemicals in food pack-aging on communities that lack access to fresh food – an environmental justice issue.* The Unwrapped Project. Retrieved July 21, 2022, from https://static1. squarespace.com/static/5f218f677f1fdb38f06cebcb/t/606f4f44d9e7f1748 004353f/1617907525433/The+Disproportionate+Impacts+of+Che+mi-cals+in+Food+Packaging+on+Communities+that+Lack+Access+to+-Fresh+Food+–+an+Environmental+Justice+Issue+%281%29.pdf

333 U.S. Food and Drug Administration. (2016, September 2). *FDA issues final rule on safety and effectiveness of antibacterial soaps.* Retrieved July 21, 2022, from https://www.fda.gov/news-events/press-announcements/ fda-issues-final-rule-safety-and-effectiveness-antibacterial-soaps

334 USDA. (2002, May 15). *Spray weeds with vinegar?* Retrieved July 21, 2022, from https://www.ars.usda.gov/news-events/news/research-news/2002/ spray-weeds-with-vinegar/

335 Environmental Working Group. (2005, July 14). *Body burden: The pol-lution in newborns.* Retrieved July 21, 2022, from https://www.ewg.org/ research/body-burden-pollution-newborns

OTHER BOOKS BY PETER KOZLOWSKI, MD

UNFUNC YOUR GUT: *A Functional Medicine Guide:*
Boost Your Immune System, Heal Your Gut and
Unlock Your Mental, Emotional and Spiritual Health
Featuring **THE KOZ PLAN:**
50+ Elimination Diet Recipes with Low-FODMAP Options

AUDIOBOOKS

UNFUNC YOUR GUT
GET THE FUNC OUT

ABOUT THE AUTHOR

As a Functional Medicine MD, Dr. Peter Kozlowski uses a broad array of tools to find the source of the body's dysfunction: he takes the time to listen to his patients and plots their history on a timeline, considering what makes them unique and co-creating with them a truly individualized care plan. A graduate of Family Medicine Residency, he has devoted his career to helping uncover the underlying cause of chronic disease through Functional Medicine. He trained with leaders in his field including Dr. Mark Hyman, Dr. Deepak Chopra, and Dr. Susan Blum. His bestselling health and diet book, *Unfunc Your Gut,* was named the winner of International Book Awards. He serves patients in person and online via his Montana- and Chicago-based practices.

www.doc-koz.com

PUBLISHER'S NOTE

Thank you for the opportunity to serve you. If you would like to help share this message, here are some popular ways:

- **Reviews:** Write an online book review

- **Giving:** Gift this book to friends, family, and colleagues

- **Book Clubs:** Read it with a group of friends, discuss your experiences, and prepare *Koz Plan* recipes (from Doc Koz's first book, *Unfunc Your Gut)* for your meeting

- **Book Tour:** Suggest your city or hometown as a stop: booktours@citrinepublishing.com

- **Speaking:** Invite Doc Koz to speak with your organization via www.doc-koz.com

- **Workshops:** Request an *Unfunc Your Gut* or *Get the Func Out* workshop in your area via www.doc-koz.com

- **Bulk Orders:** Email sales@citrinepublishing.com

- **Contact Information:** Call +1-828-585-7030 or email: info@citrinepublishing.com

We appreciate your book reviews, letters, and shares.

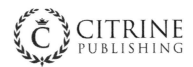

CITRINE PUBLISHING

Made in United States
Troutdale, OR
06/14/2023